THE · BUSINESS ·  PRACTICE

Making Sense of Practice Finance

Third Edition

Edited by
JOHN DEAN

Foreword by
JOHN CHISHOLM

RADCLIFFE MEDICAL PRESS

Radcliffe Medical Press Ltd
18 Marcham Road, Abingdon, Oxon OX14 1AA

First edition 1990
Second edition 1994

British Library Cataloguing in Publication Data

A catalogue record for this book is available from the British Library.

ISBN 1 85775 331 3

Typeset by Advance Typesetting Ltd, Oxon
Printed and bound by TJ International Ltd, Padstow, Cornwall

Contents

Foreword

General practitioners, as independent contractors, are responsible not only for the clinical care they provide to patients, but also for the organisation and finances of their practices. Young doctors entering general practice may have been attracted by the variety of patients, the prospects for continuing care and the practice of whole-person medicine, but they soon discover that they must also acquire the administration skills needed to run a small business with a substantial turnover. Without those skills, they will fail the patients they seek to serve and the staff they employ and they will fail also to maximise their income.

Developments in the 1990s have emphasised the importance of value for money and increased the need for organisational and financial discipline. This book is intended to meet that need. It should be essential reading for every GP and will also be useful for practice managers, practice accountants and GP registrars.

John Dean and the other contributors to this third edition of *Making Sense of Practice Finance* are all experts in their fields and John is renowned as one of the leading authorities in the highly specialised and complex area of general practice taxation and accountancy. The first two editions of this book proved to be a vital reference document and this considerably expanded and updated new edition will, I am sure, prove even more valuable.

JOHN CHISHOLM
Chairman
General Medical Services Committee
British Medical Association
December 1999

Preface

The success of the first two editions of *Making Sense of Practice Finance* demonstrated the degree to which GPs have in recent years become far more conscious of their finances. It is no longer acceptable for them, and for young GPs with financial obligations in particular, to be content to run their practices as clinical organisations only, with little regard for their earnings levels.

During the 1990s there has been tremendous growth in the income of medical practices, some of this arising through the effects of GP fund-holding and some from the effects of the 1990 GP Contract. The typical medical practice is no longer a 'cottage industry' run from a private house of the doctor. Instead, there is a trend towards larger practices, higher levels of earnings and a far more businesslike approach than has been seen in the past. The practice with a turnover in excess of £1 million, which in the 1980s was exceptional, is now relatively commonplace.

All this means that GPs, although delegating much of their management and administrative functions to practice managers and other highly qualified staff, must remain aware of the manner in which they are paid, how their income is taxed, how their income tax will be settled and the numerous financial problems arising in partnerships.

Since the second edition was published in 1994 there have been major changes in the manner in which income is taxed. The introduction of the current-year basis of assessment and self-assessment for taxpayers has come as something of a rude shock to those who were never efficient in submitting tax returns, supplying income for completion of accounts and the like. The ending of the GP fundholding scheme is another major change and has radically affected the finances of many former fundholding practices.

For the sake of brevity and to avoid the use of contorted English, it has been assumed throughout that all GPs are male and all practice managers female. Although this is manifestly not the case, readers are invited to convert this to their own situations as necessary.

Any reference to the finances of individual practices, or doctors, is purely for example and bears no relation to any known practices. This particularly applies to the specimen accounts set out in Chapter 10, whose sole purpose is to provide points of reference for explanations of accounting procedures in this and other chapters.

While every effort has been made during the preparation of this book to ensure that information is as up to date as possible, readers should bear in mind that fees and allowances, tax rates and particularly interest rates can change at relatively short notice. In making any decisions based on the information in this book, up-to-date advice should always be sought.

The preparation of this new edition would not have been possible without the assistance of contributors and specialist colleagues who have helped both by making contributions and in reviewing the content at various stages.

JOHN DEAN
December 1999

About the editor

John Dean is a Certified Public Accountant who has specialised in the financial taxation and accountancy affairs of members of the medical profession for over 20 years. He is accepted as a leading authority on the subject and is in considerable demand as a lecturer to doctors, GP registrars, practice managers and accountants.

John also writes extensively for medical and dental journals. His first book, *Making Sense of Practice Finance*, was first published in 1990, with a second edition in 1994. *Practice Finance: your questions answered* was first published by Radcliffe Medical Press in 1992, with a second edition in 1998.

A series of publications essentially aimed at the accountancy profession is published by Accountancy Books.

As Director of Medical Services with a national firm of chartered accountants, John set up his own business during 1993. Since 1999 he has been a partner in the specialist accounting firm of Dean Taylor Associates.

From 1995 to 1997, he was founder chairman of the Association of Independent Specialist Medical Accountants (AISMA).

List of contributors

Malcolm Dalley is the principal of Seabrook Investment Services Ltd and has been in the financial services business for over 20 years, much of which has been spent advising members of the medical profession. He is also a member of the Society of Financial Advisers.

Norman Ellis is Under Secretary at the British Medical Association. His own books include *Making Sense of the Red Book* (3rd edition), *General Practice Employment Handbook* and *General Practitioners' Handbook* (2nd edition), all published by Radcliffe Medical Press.

Michael Gilbert is a chartered accountant, well known as a specialist in the field of GP finance. He is chairman of the Association of Independent Specialist Medical Accountants.

John Lindsay is head of the Superannuation Department at the BMA. His books include *Staff Pensions in General Practice* (Radcliffe Medical Press).

Michael North is a partner in Messrs Clarkson, Wright & Jakes, Solicitors of Orpington, who specialise in work for medical practitioners, including the settlement of partnership disputes and preparation of partnership deeds.

Ray Stanbridge is a practising accountant and business adviser with his own firm of financial management consultants, Stanbridge Associates Ltd.

Terry Taylor is a Certified Public Accountant and a partner in Dean Taylor Associates. He has specialised in the accountancy affairs of GPs for some fifteen years.

List of abbreviations

AVC	additional voluntary contributions
BMA	British Medical Association
BPA	basic practice allowance
CGT	capital gains tax
DoH	Department of Health
DTI	Department of Trade and Industry
EU	European Union
FIMBRA	Financial Intermediaries, Managers and Brokers Regulatory Association
FSAVC	free-standing additional voluntary contribution
GMC	General Medical Council
GMP	general medical practice/practitioner
GMSC	General Medical Services Committee (of the BMA)
GP	general practitioner
HA	health authority
HPC	health promotion committee
IHT	inheritance tax
ISA	individual saving account(s)
LMC	local medical committee
MMR	mumps, measles and rubella
NHSPS	NHS pension scheme
NIC	National Insurance contributions
PAYE	pay-as-you-earn tax
PCG	Primary Care Group
PEP	personal equity plan
PGEA	postgraduate education allowance
PIA	personal investment authority
RCGP	Royal College of General Practitioners
SFA	statement of fees and allowances (the Red Book)
SMP	statutory maternity pay
SSP	statutory sick pay
TESSA	tax-exempt special savings account
VAT	value added tax

1 Fees and allowances
Norman Ellis

Where to obtain advice and assistance
Help can be obtained from the HA/Health Board and LMC offices. BMA
members can also contact their local BMA office for advice and assistance.

Further reading includes Ellis N and Chisholm J (1997) *Making Sense of
the Red Book* (3e). Radcliffe Medical Press, Oxford.

The GPs' pay system is particularly complex and hard to understand. GPs
earn their income from a range of fees and allowances. These are of four
broad types: fixed allowances, capitation-based payments, item-of-service
payments and bonus payments. They are set each year at levels which will
both yield the finite 'pool' of money available to fund GPs' net income and
meet those expenses not reimbursed directly by the HA or Health Board.
The 'pool' which funds GPs' net income is calculated by multiplying average intended net remuneration by the number of GP principals.

If the relative level of any fee or allowance is altered (e.g. by increasing
the basic practice allowance or decreasing capitation fees), the remaining
fees and allowances are changed so that the total amount of money paid out
to GPs remains at the right level. Unless additional funds are specifically
made available by government (colloquially known as 'new money'), according to the current pay system it is not possible to increase any specific fees
or allowances without simultaneously reducing some other fee(s) so as to
maintain the level of net remuneration.

This chapter outlines the main fees and allowances payable to GPs which
were newly introduced or substantially modified by the 1990 contract and
subsequent additions. Full details of all fees and allowances are given in
the Statement of Fees and Allowances (otherwise known as the SFA or Red
Book). Current GMS fees and allowances are set out in Appendix A.

Basic practice allowance

GPs qualify for the basic practice allowance (BPA) if their individual list
size or partnership average list size is at least 400 patients; a GP with at
least 400 patients is paid a BPA and its level increases with list size up to a
ceiling of 1200 patients. Thus a lump sum is paid for the first 400 patients

and additional capitation payments are then made for each patient between 400 and 600, 600 and 800, 800 and 1000, and 1000 and 1200. By weighting the level of these capitation payments in favour of the lower list size, the BPA is designed to compensate for the proportionately greater standing expenses incurred by a small practice than a larger one. The BPA is also weighted in favour of part-time GPs; that of a half-time GP is significantly greater than half that of a full-time GP.

Deprivation payments

GPs are paid a capitation-based supplement to the BPA, known as the 'deprivation payment', for all patients living within an area classified as 'deprived' according to the Jarman deprivation index, whether or not the individual or family is actually deprived. This supplement is intended to reflect the higher workload associated with some categories of patients. GPs with individual or average partnership lists of less than 400 patients who are not paid a BPA nevertheless qualify for deprivation payments for patients living in deprived areas. There are three levels of payment according to the degree of deprivation (as measured by the Jarman index) of the area where the patient lives.

Seniority awards

Principals in general practice receive payment in recognition of length of service. The scales and thresholds for payment changed in 1999 with, for the first time, the introduction of a fourth stage payment.

There are three levels of seniority payment:

- the first level is paid to a GP registered for 10 years and providing general medical services for at least 6 years
- the second level is paid to a GP registered for 17 years or more and providing general medical services for at least 13 years
- the third level is paid to a GP registered for 23 years or more and providing general medical services for at least 19 years
- the fourth level is paid to a GP registered for 29 years or more and providing general medical services for at least 25 years.

This fourth level of payment was introduced only with effect from 1 April 1999.

Payments, reduced proportionately, are made to part-time GPs and those full-time GPs not eligible for the full BPA. Job-sharers are assessed for the seniority payment on an individual basis and payment is reduced according to their hours of availability.

Within partnerships, a decision has to be made as to whether a partner will retain his seniority award personally or whether this will be pooled with the residue of partnership profits for division. In the vast majority of medical partnerships it is agreed that principals will retain their seniority themselves, effectively this being credited to them through the partnership accounts as a prior share of profit.

Capitation fees

The standard capitation fees are paid at three rates according to a patient's age: under 65 years, 65–74 years, and 75 years and over.

Registration fee

This is paid to a GP who carries out certain health checks on a newly registered patient (except those aged under five years), normally within three months of joining the list. As with seniority awards, in many cases, these will be allocated to the partners in whose names they are paid. This will affect the allocation of profits where the partners do not share profits equally. PGEA will invariably be treated through the partnership accounts as a prior share of profits.

Postgraduate education allowance

The postgraduate education allowance (PGEA) is paid to any GP who undertakes a programme of continuing education; it is intended to cover any course fees, travel and subsistence costs.

To receive the full rate of the PGEA, GPs must demonstrate to their HA/ Health Board that they have attended an average of five days' training a year over the past five years. Although the amount of time spent on courses may vary from year to year, a GP is expected to achieve a reasonable balance between years. Courses are divided into three areas:

- health promotion and prevention of illness
- disease management
- service management.

To claim the PGEA, GPs have to attend at least two courses under each of the three subject areas over the five years preceding the claim. The length of course is not actually defined in the Red Book; postgraduate deans have discretion to determine what constitutes a 'course' for the purpose of completing a balanced educational programme.

A GP should claim the allowance from the HA/Health Board each year, giving details of courses attended over the five-year period. Any GP who meets the required criteria (25 days' training and at least two courses under each of the three headings) is paid a full PGEA in quarterly instalments. Lower levels of the allowance are paid if courses are spread across only one or two of the subject areas or less than the maximum length of training is undertaken.

Target payments for childhood immunisation and cervical cytology

In 1990 the government introduced target payments for childhood immunisation and cervical cytology. There are two levels of payment. For childhood immunisation, a higher level of payment is made to GPs who achieve 90% coverage and a lower level for 70% coverage. For cervical cancer screening the upper level is 80% and the lower 50%. These are calculated on a partnership basis.

Childhood immunisation

There are two target levels, 70% and 90%, and these relate to average coverage levels across four groups of immunisations:

- Group I   – diphtheria, tetanus and poliomyelitis
- Group II – pertussis
- Group III – mumps, measles and rubella (MMR)
- Group IV – haemophilius influenzae type B (Hib).

A target is reached if, on average across the four groups, 70% or 90% of the children aged two years on a GP's list have had complete courses of immunisation (i.e. three doses of diphtheria, tetanus and poliomyelitis, or three doses of pertussis, or one dose of MMR, or three doses of Hib). To calculate this, the coverage level in each group is taken into account and the mean of these is the overall coverage level. For example, if a practice has ten children on the list aged two years all of whom have had complete courses of diphtheria, tetanus, poliomyelitis and Hib, nine who have had a complete course of pertussis and eight who have had the MMR immunisation, the overall coverage level is nine out of ten, that is 90%. Thus, the higher target level has been reached. All complete immunisation courses count towards coverage levels whether done by the GP making the claim or some other person, such as a community health clinic doctor.

The maximum payment a GP can receive depends on how many children aged two years are on the list; the Red Book describes how this is calculated. The proportion of the maximum payment made to a GP reflects the amount of this work done within general medical services, rather than in a clinic or hospital setting, whether in the patient's current practice or a previous one. Thus, if the 90% level is achieved, and GPs have done 70% of all the complete courses of immunisation, the claiming GP receives 7/9 of the maximum payment.

Pre-school boosters for children under five years

Again, there are two target levels: 70% and 90%. A target is reached if at least 70% or 90% of children aged five years on a GP's list have had reinforcing doses of diphtheria, tetanus and poliomyelitis immunisations. The arrangements for calculating these payments are similar to those described above.

Cervical cytology

There are two target levels: 50% and 80%; a target is reached if 50% or 80% of women on a GP's list aged 25–64 years in England and Wales (or aged 21–60 years in Scotland) have had an adequate cervical smear test during the previous 5.5 years. (This period is based on a five-year call/recall system with an allowance for unavoidable delays.) All smear tests are counted, not just those taken in general practice. For the purpose of calculating coverage, women who have had hysterectomies (involving the complete removal of the cervix) are excluded.

The maximum size of the target payment a GP can receive depends on the number of eligible women on the list. The actual proportion of the maximum payment paid to a GP reflects the work done by GPs (and their staff) as opposed to others, such as the private sector and community health services.

Child health surveillance fee

To be paid for child health surveillance GPs must be on the HA/Health Board child health surveillance list; admission to this requires them to satisfy the criteria relating to experience and training set out in the regulations. A capitation supplement is paid for each child patient under the age of five years to whom a GP provides developmental surveillance, if the child is registered with the GP for this purpose.

Minor surgery payments

A sessional payment is made to GPs on the HA/Health Board minor surgery list who personally provide minor surgery services. A session consists of at least five surgical procedures, performed either in a single clinic or on separate occasions. GPs can undertake minor surgery for patients on their own personal list or that of a partner or another member of the group practice. A GP is eligible for no more than three such payments in respect of any one quarter. However, a GP who is in a partnership or group may claim additional payments, provided the total number of payments to the partnership or group per quarter does not exceed three times the number of GPs involved. Up to four minor surgery procedures can be carried forward for inclusion in the following quarter's claim.

Night consultation fees and night allowance

All GPs are paid an annual night allowance in partial recognition of their 24-hour responsibility for patients. This allowance is paid at a flat rate per GP with job sharers counting as a single GP for this purpose.

In addition GPs are paid a fee for each face-to-face consultation requested and undertaken between 10 p.m. and 8 a.m. with a patient who is:

- on their list of patients
- a temporary resident
- a woman for whom they had undertaken to provide maternity medical services in connection with which the consultation is provided.

Where the GP is separately engaged or employed by an NHS trust or HA to provide services in any premises owned or managed by the trust or authority, the fee is paid only if the GP is not on duty or on call at those premises and the request for the patient to be seen was made in accordance with paragraph 13 of the terms of service. However, if the GP visits the patient in a hospital to provide maternity medical services, a consultation fee is paid if he holds an appointment at the hospital, but was not on duty at the time, or if he does not hold such an appointment in respect of maternity medical services.

The fee is paid to the GP with whom the patient is registered, regardless of whether the visit is made by:

- the GP with whom the patient is registered
- a partner or another GP from the practice
- an assistant, associate, GP registrar, locum or deputy employed by the partnership or group, or a doctor in the same out-of-hours rota.

Associate allowance

Single-handed GPs in very isolated areas (e.g. the Highlands and Islands) are eligible for an associate allowance, enabling them, in conjunction with other single-handed GPs, to employ an associate GP who can provide services for patients during absences for social and professional purposes.

Health promotion payments

A new payment system based on practices developing their own health promotion programmes was introduced in October 1996. The new scheme is based on a single level of payment for health promotion activities approved by local, professionally led, health promotion committees. The amount a practice receives is related to list size.

Activities must relate to:

- modern authoritative medical opinion
- the Health of the Nation strategy and/or
- patient needs and/or
- local health priorities.

There are separate payments for organising chronic disease management programmes for either asthma or diabetes. These require practices to develop guidelines for delivering care to these patients.

Other fees and allowances

- additions to the BPA for employing an assistant
- inducement payments
- initial practice allowances
- mileage payments
- temporary resident fees

- fees for emergency treatment
- fees for immediately necessary treatment
- fees for maternity medical services
- fees for contraceptive services
- fees for public policy vaccinations and immunisations
- fees for service as an anaesthetist and for arresting a dental haemorrhage
- payments for supplying drugs and appliances
- payments during sickness and confinement – there are no list size restrictions for employing a locum during confinement
- locum allowances for single-handed practitioners in rural areas attending educational courses
- prolonged study leave allowance
- trainee practitioner scheme payments
- doctors' retainer scheme payments
- payments under the rent and rates scheme
- improvement grants
- payments under the practice staff scheme
- payments under the computer reimbursement scheme.

Claiming correct fees and allowances

The NHS GPs' remuneration system is probably the most complex in the world. It takes several hundred pages and an estimated 350 000 words of the regulations and the Red Book to determine how and what a GP should be paid. Every practice should ensure that it is claiming correct fees and allowances, otherwise it will not receive its correct remuneration. Conversely, no claim should ever be made, whether knowingly or unknowingly, for a fee or allowance to which a GP or practice is not entitled. False or improper claims can have very serious consequences; HAs have not hesitated to instigate criminal proceedings against GPs who have made such unjustified claims.

2 Other income sources

NHS general practice generates, in most cases, the majority of its income from the HA by means of GMS fees, allowances and the various available refunds as outlined in Chapter 1.

However, there is nothing to stop GPs, either personally or through their partnership, from earning additional income; indeed the vast majority of general practices do so to a greater or lesser degree.

The extent to which these other income sources apply to any given practice normally depends on such items as the nature of the locality and patients, the philosophy of the GPs and the commitment the partners are prepared to give to the practice. Nevertheless, such income is a useful and regular supplement for practices and frequently makes the difference between an averagely remunerated practice and one in which the partners are receiving incomes well above published levels.

Fees received by many practices include the following:

1 *Insurance reports and medicals.* Most practices receive a fairly regular source of income from reports and, in some cases, examinations on behalf of insurance companies which require information concerning the health of patients taking out life assurance policies. For expensive policies a particularly rigorous examination may be required.
2 *Public service medicals.* Many practices receive regular payments for such items as attendance allowances or civil service medicals for certain patients. In some cases, GPs are appointed by a local public office to deal with such medicals and are paid separately from that source.
3 *Examinations and procedures on behalf of patients.* A steady but modest income can be earned from such items as HGV medicals for drivers, completion of BUPA referral forms, passport applications and numerous other items. Some GPs are uncertain about the fees they should charge for such work. Suggested fees are published on a regular basis, both in medical journals and by the BMA. A notice should be placed in the reception area or waiting room so that patients can see the cost of such services.
4 *Cremation fees.* Many GPs receive income from signing cremation certificates and a fee is obtained for this. It is important that this is

properly recorded and shown separately in the practice accounts. This is because the Inland Revenue can (and does) send representatives to examine the books of undertakers and crematoria to obtain details of fees paid to GPs. The Inland Revenue is then able to cross-check with the GPs' accounts to see if these have been properly returned. Failure to do so has proved expensive for some practices and can lead, in extreme cases, to a full examination of the GPs' accounts, with potentially disastrous consequences.

5 *Police surgeon fees.* Some GPs are appointed police doctors and are called to the scene of accidents to perform breathalyser tests, etc. For a practice that obtains such an appointment on a regular basis, the income received can be significant, although this is offset by the unsocial hours often required.

6 *Company medicals and retainers.* Some GPs obtain appointments with local businesses. The work can be extensive, looking after the medical affairs of a large workforce. On the other hand, it may require only occasional attendance. In many cases, a retainer can be obtained which will give a regular source of income.

7 *Sundry cash fees.* It is important that any cash fees received in the surgery, for sundry certificates, passports or sick notes, are properly recorded and paid to the bank at regular intervals. If retained personally by the GPs, they must be declared to the Inland Revenue (*see* Chapter 9) through the self-assessment tax returns of the doctors concerned.

8 *Private patients.* Many practices attract private patients. This depends primarily on the locality and to some extent on the practice policy. Some practices discourage private patients for reasons of conscience. If private patients are accepted, they should be dealt with in a businesslike manner; accounts should be rendered at regular intervals, normally monthly or in some cases quarterly, and procedures should be instituted to ensure that payment is received with minimum delay. For larger private practices, a more complete credit control system may be required.

9 *Hospital appointments.* Some practices obtain appointments at local hospitals as clinical assistants, casualty officers or for attendances at clinics. These part-time hospital appointments are normally taxed and care must be taken to see that the fees are paid into the practice account if that is the policy of the partnership. Earnings from appointments at local hospitals may be taxed at source, which can cause a problem in partnerships (*see* Chapter 23).

10 *Co-operatives.* Many GPs are now members of local co-operative organisations, which deal with the provision of night visits and out-of-hours

facilities. In many cases, partnerships will arrange for partners who choose to deal with work of this nature to receive the income themselves, rather than to pay this into the partnership pool. Care must be taken to ensure these are properly accounted for, as indicated below, and assessed correctly for tax purposes. In many cases also, the local co-operative will provide each year a statement setting out the notional amount earned by the practice, but which is offset by matching expenditure. Although no cash will pass, nevertheless the total of such a figure should be passed through on both sides of the accounts in order to ensure that expenditure is maximised, possibly for Review Body purposes.

Partnership earnings

The partnership deed should define what are and what are not partnership earnings. This will depend on the policy of the partnership, but it should nevertheless be clearly set out in the deed.

Well-organised partnerships, operating with a high level of financial discipline, usually insist that all medical earnings of the partners, from whatever source, are paid into the partnership account for division between the partners in agreed ratios. Failure to do so can give rise to disputes between partners.

Where, exceptionally, partnerships agree to divide certain amounts of these earnings in a manner other than in which partnership profits are shared, then these should also be treated as a prior share of profits.

Accounting problems

Provided that all income of this nature is properly recorded within the partnership accounts, paid to the bank and properly treated for tax purposes, few, if any, problems will arise. Cash receipts should *not* be treated as a float out of which petty cash expenditure can be made (*see* Chapter 9).

All practices should have in force a methodical system of recording income of this nature; ensuring that, whether by cheque or in cash, all such receipts are paid regularly into the bank account and are correctly treated for tax purposes.

Where it is accepted that some partners will retain some or all of these earnings, then the partner concerned should ensure that income retained by him by those means is properly recorded and included each year in his self-assessment tax return.

Primary care groups

At 31 March 1999, fundholding ceased to operate for the provision of primary care services. This was replaced by primary care groups, or PCGs.

The purpose of primary care groups is to implement policies and primary care services for a wide range of practices, each operating within a given area, rather than have individual practices implementing their individual policies and services.

As far as practice finance is concerned, this has a number of significant impacts. Firstly, the control for funding of budgets is no longer undertaken by each practice, but instead this is operated by the PCG. Secondly, practices no longer receive an allowance for the increased costs of implementing these budgets. Instead, these costs are controlled by the PCG. Thirdly, PCGs are run by a number of groups from society, of which the most significant is, quite rightly, GPs. Only a select few GPs are able to become significantly involved in the management of a PCG, and the funding for their time is in the form of either a fee or salary, the level of which is dependent upon the status of the GP. The GP who is involved in the PCG management will either be a Board Member, or Chairperson of a Board. The Chairperson receives a higher scale than the board member.

Practices will need to determine whether the earnings from the PCG boards should be treated as practice income for division in profit-sharing ratios, or whether the individual doctor should be able to retain this money personally. As with all GP earnings, it is better that the funds pass through the practice account, whether or not the individual partner will retain the fee.

As far as the demise of fundholding is concerned, it will be necessary to closely monitor expenditure, to ensure that previously reimbursed costs are no longer being incurred.

3 Claiming direct refunds

A range of expenses paid directly by GPs for their practices are reimbursed directly to them, wholly or in part, by the HA. It is important that the procedure for making a claim is understood, to ensure that full refunds are received. It is also necessary for such expenditure to be grossed up in the accounts so that expenses are maximised in the event of their being examined as part of the Review Body sampling process.

General practice is the only profession, inside or outside the NHS, that has this extremely beneficial system of direct refunds, by which GPs are effectively 'cushioned' against rises in expenditure during times of high inflation and periods of low pay increases. High-cost items, such as rates and trainees' salaries, will normally be repaid in full.

It is, however, surprising how many practices fail to benefit fully from this system, usually because of inadequate claiming procedures, which have lost practices many thousands of pounds.

All practices should therefore set up an efficient system for claiming these refunds. Where possible, responsibility for this should be delegated to the practice manager or one of her staff, who will be responsible for ensuring that correct claims are submitted and that accurate refunds are obtained from the HA. The SFA is the definitive reference and should be consulted when doubt arises. Relevant paragraphs in the SFA follow.

Rents

Paragraph 51. Where a practice rents a surgery from a third party, i.e. a landlord, the rent paid is normally reimbursed in full. However, in some cases GPs do not use the whole of the leased building for NHS purposes; in such cases a restriction is applied and only a proportion of the rent is reimbursable. Where this applies, the district valuer visits the premises and assesses the proportion of rent qualifying for refund.

The district valuer may consider the rent paid to be above the market rental value of the property, in which case a lower notional rent figure may be substituted. GPs do not, therefore, have a 'carte blanche' facility to pay out, and be refunded, an unlimited amount in rent. The amount paid must always be relevant both to the level of accommodation provided and known rental values.

GPs who own their own surgeries receive either a notional or cost rent allowance (*see* Chapter 15).

Rates

Paragraph 51.13(b). GPs can claim a full refund of all rates paid on behalf of their surgeries. This normally includes:

• uniform business rates
• water rates
• water (metered) charges (paragraph 51.13(c))
• drainage rates
• sewerage rates.

The latter two items apply only in some areas. In some urban areas a charge may be made by the local authority for disposal of trade refuse. Where this occurs, a refund should be claimed from the HA (paragraph 51.13(d)). Rates will not be reimbursed where the rental includes a charge for rates.

Some practices choose to make payments of business rates by monthly standing orders, normally by ten such payments between April and January each year. Care must be taken to see that these instalments are recovered on a regular basis, which is normally quarterly.

In some areas, HAs have agreed to make payments of this nature, normally business and water rates, direct to the local authority or water company concerned, without any cash passing through the practice. This is attractive to practices who consequently do not have to concern themselves with making payments or dealing with the claiming and receipt of the refund. However, it does impose on the practice an obligation to ensure that these figures are included on both sides of the accounts (*see* Chapter 10). The mere fact that they are not passed physically through the accounts does not mean they can be ignored.

Ancillary staff refunds

Until the mid-1990s it was common for practices to be refunded 70% of the gross salaries of all ancillary staff and 100% of the employer's share of the National Insurance contribution. However, this is no longer normally the case as payments are now subject to negotiation with the HA.

For the practice to qualify for a refund, ancillary staff may be engaged to carry out certain duties:

- nursing and treatment
- secretarial and clerical work, including records and filing
- receiving patients
- making appointments
- dispensing.

It should be noted that this scheme does not include salaries of cleaners, which do not qualify for a refund. Salaries of practice managers are generally held to fall within the qualifying parameters. Salaries paid to GPs' spouses also normally qualify for a refund (*see* Chapter 26). Moreover, staff engaged in a wider range of duties – including physiotherapists, dietitians, counsellors, link workers, translators, etc. – may also now qualify.

The system has changed significantly over recent years, as HAs must now impose cash limits on refunds of this nature. Practices should try to negotiate with the HA beforehand to ensure that their ancillary staff refund is maximised.

Where such cash limits are imposed, however, some HAs quote a standard figure for the ensuing year, which is paid in monthly instalments, regardless of the number of staff engaged by that particular practice. Different considerations do, however, apply in various parts of the country and practices should be aware of the policy of their own HA.

For example, a practice and HA may agree that the annual budget for ancillary staff refunds in a year is £70 000. For this to represent a standard recovery rate on a gross amount of salaries paid, the practice should try to so organise its affairs that the total salary bill in a typical year, for qualified ancillary staff only, comes to no more than about £100 000. This would represent a recovery rate of 70% but effectively ignores the fact that the practice should also seek to recover 100% of the employer's National Insurance contributions (*see* Chapter 28). An ideal recovery rate, if the practice can possibly be so organised, would be in the range of 71–72%.

GPs in health centres

Paragraph 53. There is normally no direct charge for rent and rates to doctors practising from publicly owned health centres (normally owned and administered by the HA).

Instead the payments are usually dealt with internally, without passing through the practice bank account. In such cases, it is important that the figure for rent or rates be obtained and included as an item of both expense and refund on both sides of the annual practice accounts. This serves the purpose of maximising expenses in case the accounts are required for examination by the Review Body.

Similarly, some practices in health centres do not employ their own staff; they are administered and paid by the HA. In such cases, the doctor is normally charged a net percentage of staff salaries, with a full remission of National Insurance contributions (NIC). Again, it is necessary for this expenditure to be grossed up, in the case of salaries with 100% shown on the expenditure side and the appropriate percentage as a refund. NIC should also be shown fully on both sides of the accounts. This information should be automatically supplied to the practice at regular intervals.

In some areas, the practice has grown in the last few years of asking practices to pay a rental charge for their Health Centre accommodation, which is then recovered from the HA as with other direct refunds. Again, care must be taken to ensure that a 100% refund will be obtained.

GP registrars

GPs who undertake the training of young doctors are paid a fee in the form of a trainee supervision grant.

For practice purposes, the GP registrar, during his year with the practice, is paid a salary based on a scale negotiated from time to time and advised to the practice by the HA. This salary is paid to the trainee as if he were a normal employee of the practice, with the full range of pay-as-you-earn (PAYE) and Class 1 NI deductions being imposed.

A refund is, however, made to the practice of the amount of the gross salary, plus the car allowance, medical defence body subscription and the employer's share of the NIC.

Training practices are dealt with in more detail in Chapter 17.

Car parking

In some urban areas, where it is necessary for the doctors to use a municipal car park, a refund of car-parking charges can be claimed from the HA under a local agreement. This is normally in the form of a refund of fees charged for contract parking tickets. In some cases a similar arrangement will apply in respect of staff parking charges.

Drug refunds

Many practices make claims for repayment of the costs of drugs dispensed or prescribed for patients. GPs should ensure that they make their claims on a regular basis. Refunds are normally made in arrears, often by as much as three months. Dispensing practices are dealt with in more detail in Chapter 18.

Computer grants

Paragraph 58. A scheme is in force whereby GPs can obtain a refund of part of the cost of installing computers in their practice, as well as for leasing and maintenance costs.

Payments on account

GPs can obtain by right monthly payments on account of many of the items described in this chapter, except rates (unless paid by monthly standing order) or rent, which are normally repaid on presentation of the necessary receipt. It is particularly important in respect of ancillary staff and trainee refunds that payments on account are received monthly, with a balance at the end of the quarter. If properly done, this could have a significant effect on the practice's cash flow position.

In all cases, care should be taken to ensure that refunds are claimed in an efficient and systematic manner, to ensure a prompt flow of cash through the practice. The responsibility for claiming refunds lies entirely with the practice, and it is not unusual to find practices failing to claim some or all of the items described, with significant effects on the earning levels of the partners.

A well drawn up set of practice accounts should show that refunds have been obtained, and the payment on one side should match the refund obtained on the other (*see* Chapter 10).

Abatement of direct refunds

The SFA in paragraphs 51.16 and 52.19 authorises HAs to make a deduction or abatement from direct refunds in certain cases where it can be shown that fees from non-NHS sources amount to more than 10% of the gross practice income. Where two surgeries are in use, this percentage increases to 15%. Gross practice income is not clearly defined, but it is generally considered to represent the total income of the practice from all sources, including refunds, but excluding income from NHS sources other than that received via the HA, such as earnings from hospital appointments. The illustration of gross practice income, in the specimen accounts on pages 62–77 is from an example practice with a total income from all sources of £582 492. Any possible abatement of refunds would, for that example, be calculated as follows.

	Total income (£)	Non-NHS income (£)
Gross income, per accounts	582 492	
Income from appointments (Note 11)		61 466
Non-NHS fees (Note 12)		12 478
		73 944
Less: Interest, etc.	(1246)	
NHS appointments		
(Note 11): £9648 + £2645	(12 293)	(12 293)
	568 953	61 651

The proportion of non-NHS income using this formula is 10.8%, so the practice may suffer abatement of direct refunds. It should be noted, however, that this rule only applies to the use of wholly or partially financed NHS premises or staff for private purposes. The proceeds from non-NHS work carried out, for example at the GP's home, can be omitted from the calculation.

In the case of the practice illustrated in Chapter 10, from which the above calculation derives (Note 11; page 70), a high proportion of the non-NHS income comes from work as a police surgeon. Therefore, provided the practice can convince the HA that NHS-financed premises or staff are not used for this purpose, it should not suffer abatement.

4 Management and efficiency in general practice

It has been said, perhaps to the point of repetition, that efficiency is an attitude of mind. In the same way also, it is rare that a leopard changes its spots, and fortunate indeed is the inefficient practice which, possibly by engagement of a new practice manager, transforms itself into an efficient practice, properly managed and highly profitable. Perhaps in no other profession is efficient financial management so productive in terms of the eventual outcome – the net disposable incomes of the partners.

Not only will this affect the partners who, being the key professionals involved, display their knowledge and skills in earning such a level of income, but also the other members of the primary healthcare team whose support and effort are equally essential.

In general medical practice, this can be immediately seen where the financial results of differing practices are compared. It is by no means unusual to find apparently otherwise identical practices turning in vastly different financial results and, hence, the income of the partners.

General practice is as much a business as the work of professionals outside the healthcare field, such as that of solicitors, accountants or architects, who sell their professional skills with a view to profit. In the same way, the profitable business is likely to be the financially efficient one.

Discrepancies in income levels in general practice are by no means unusual. On the one hand, one may find a highly efficient dispensing or training practice, with several outside appointments, some private patient earnings, maximum staff levels and the partners earning incomes in excess of £80 000 per annum.

Such a practice is likely to be a highly efficient, medium-sized business, with the partners all taking a share of executive responsibility and the practice manager dealing with the day-to-day running of the practice, leaving the doctors largely to concentrate on their clinical duties to the ultimate benefit of the patients.

At the other end of the scale, there may be an apparently identical practice, but where the partners take little interest in administration and operate on a shoestring, with two or three part-time receptionists, no recognisable practice manager and little attention being made to the regular submission of item-of-service claims; the lack of attention is all too evident.

Those who are privileged to see the accounts of various doctors' practices from around the country will testify to the huge differences in incomes that can occur. Invariably, the difference between two apparently identical practices in financial terms is due to the quality of the management and the manner in which income is generated.

What then do we mean by financial efficiency and how can this be obtained? In medical practice, it generally falls into several categories:

• the maximisation of income levels, generally through item-of-service fees and target payments (Chapter 1)
• the timely and accurate claiming of refunds (Chapter 3)
• adequate staffing levels
• control over expenditure levels, with proper budgeting procedures (Chapter 5)
• a well-maintained book-keeping system (Chapter 8)
• computerisation.

Each of these are discussed in some detail in the chapters indicated.

While it cannot be guaranteed that meeting these criteria will have an automatic effect on profits, the practice that gets all these right, and has the necessary will to maintain them at a high standard, has a far greater chance of attaining reasonably high income levels than one that does not.

The role of the practice manager

It is no exaggeration to say that a qualified, experienced and committed practice manager is probably the most important person in the efficiently run practice. She (or increasingly he) should be the equivalent of a company secretary, with control over the finances, administration, management and staffing of the practice below partner level. She should attend and participate in practice meetings and generally act as guide, philosopher and friend to her doctors.

The emphasis in the job title is on the word 'manager': the practice 'manager' should be the head of the practice team. Yet, in some practices the practice manager is not taken into the confidence of the doctors and is thus excluded from the ultimate management function. She is treated as little more than a superior receptionist/secretary and has little part to play in the decision-making processes. This is ultimately to the detriment of the practice.

One of the more important tasks of the practice manager is the control of the practice finances; to ensure that these are run in an efficient and systematic manner, to maximise the practice income, keep a control on expenditure and hence increase the profitability of the practice. The accurate forecasting of finance through proper cash-flow projections is essential and is set out in Chapter 6.

Good management involves successful delegation of responsibility and the manager in general practice must be prepared, where necessary, to ensure that part of her workload is delegated to more junior staff, whom it will be more cost-effective to employ for that purpose.

Many practices fall into the trap of not adequately defining the practice manager's role; she may lack a full job description – or even, in some cases, a contract of employment – and may find herself taking conflicting instructions from different partners. She will therefore feel unappreciated and unfulfilled.

At the other end of the scale, a few enlightened practices have sought to give practical recognition of the importance of the practice manager's role by elevating her to partner status. Such a step, while in principle to be welcomed, can create problems with regard to her taxation position, liability in professional negligence cases and in relations with other senior staff.

Training

The far-sighted practice will ensure that a comprehensive and progressive programme of training is in force, not only for the partners and practice manager, but for all members of staff: receptionists, nurses, secretarial and support staff. Regular courses are organised by Radcliffe Medical Press, as well as by AHCPA and AMSPAR, which can result in a recognised professional qualification.

How to increase the practice profits

There is, of course, no magic key to the generation of above-average levels of income from general practice. However, regular examination of GPs' accounts over a period can highlight a number of factors which are invariably present in the financially successful practice. A list of these is shown in Box 4.1. While all of these are unlikely to apply to every practice, they can be used as a readily available check-list against which the practice can compare its own performance and may, as a result, institute changes which will lead to a significant improvement in profitability.

It is a popular myth that high list sizes are invariably the route to high profits. Statistical results tend to confound this; invariably the partners cannot physically cater for lists of this size and have to take recourse to expensive locums and the like.

Box 4.1: Factors present in the financially successful practice

• an average or slightly above average number of patients
• efficient system for claiming refunds (*see* Chapter 3). Check all HA schedules of income and reimbursements. Follow up any discrepancies
• work minimum (26 hours) on NHS activities
• delegate to nurses, health visitors, etc. so far as possible
• make time available to take on lucrative outside appointments
• become a dispensing practice (if possible)
• all medical earnings of the partners are pooled within the partnership
• achieve Health Promotion Band 3
• do own night visits
• all partners qualify for PGEA
• do minor surgery
• partners meet regularly and plan in advance
• cash-flow forecasting system in operation (*see* Chapter 6)
• well-organised practice team
• surgery without negative equity

Statistics

General practice is one of the few professions where regular statistics are available from which the performance of the practice can be assessed; through which decisions can be taken; and, if possible, more efficient claiming procedures introduced. The question of statistics in general practice is dealt with fully in Chapter 11.

An easy life

Invariably, generation of above-average profits in general practice is a reflection on the input of the partners and the time they are prepared to devote to the practice. Many practices feel that the only way they can provide the 24-hour cover for which they are contracted is by the use of cooperatives, deputising services and the like.

This is one of the penalties doctors pay for entering general practice; the decision between earning high incomes and enjoying a more relaxed life-style. It is ultimately a choice which only they can make. An accountant or other financial adviser can point him in the right direction and make all manner of recommendations, but at the end of the day the decision rests with the individual GP.

5 Control of expenditure
Terry Taylor

Many practices have become so concerned with increasing their income, that they completely miss the point that the object of the exercise is to increase profits. The one item that is often left out of the equation is the cost of running the practice, which is frequently allowed to run out of control, without any effort being made to restrain outgoings or to limit expenditure in any way.

A great number of practices, particularly in recent years when modest pay rises have been the norm, have found that effectively their only recourse if they wish to maintain profits at an acceptable level is to radically prune their practice costs.

The matter should be discussed on a regular basis; budgets prepared and adhered to and any unduly high or unexpected amounts of expenditure examined in detail. The following example shows how one practice largely solved the problem of spiralling costs.

	Year to 30 June 1998	Year to 30 June 1999
	£	£
Gross income	405 791	430 138
Expenditure	198 946	192 468
Profit for year	206 845	237 670

This particular practice, through a drastic pruning of expenses, managed to increase its profit by 15%. However, this was at a time of low pay increases and without any guarantee that, unless rigidly controlled, costs can be maintained at a similarly low level.

Gross income rose by 6%, from £405 791 to £430 138. This is modest but acceptable, bearing in mind the financial climate in which it was realised. It is, however, in the field of expenditure saving, that the practice has made an effort that has resulted in total costs falling by 3%. Profits for the practice (with five parity partners) have risen by over £6000 per partner, over the year.

How did they achieve this? First, income was maintained at a reasonable level and this was an efficient practice that already had high earnings. The practice introduced strict budgeting procedures to control costs and the practice manager ran an efficient cash flow forecasting system. Staff salaries were pruned as far as possible, down to the level at which the practice staff budget came into force at an acceptable recovery of about 72%.

However, the most dramatic saving was in the cutting of relief service and locum fees. In the previous year, the practice had taken on a new partner, but had not utilised this additional resource to save money in the cost of employing third party doctors. The doctors brought into force a revised rota system which ensured that not only were night visit fees maximised, but payments to locums and relief services were largely dispensed with. The cash flow forecasting system ensured that drawings could be taken when funds were available and this greatly reduced bank interest charges. Other significant savings were from accountancy fees, telephone and stationery costs.

Such a dramatic result is not possible for every practice, but most practices will be able to achieve some cost savings of this nature.

Budgeting procedures

In a conventional business, which may be operated from several separate centres, the introduction of wide-ranging budgets is often a complex and time-consuming procedure. In a typical general practice, however, such difficulties should not arise. Keeping a control on outgoings is not unduly difficult, given the impetus and the co-operation of both the practice manager and the partners. Such a budget may be drawn up shortly before the start of each financial year, or as soon as the accounting records have been completed for any given year of account. It is suggested that this be done by the practice manager and agreed by the partners at the time. Budgeting should be an item on the agenda for a management meeting held at or about that time. For convenience, the budget may be drawn up for a period that coincides with the practice's accounting year. In any case, it should be approved and operational by the end of the first month of the accounting year. If, therefore, the practice accounts end in June 1999, a budget for the ensuing year should be in force by the end of July 1999.

Table 5.1 sets out a typical expenditure budget for a practice with a year end of 30 June. It shows the total budget for 1999/00, together with the actual and cumulative costs for the first two months of the year, i.e. July and August 1999, illustrating how it is possible to make a running check of expenses by this means.

It is important that not only is the budget drawn up at the proper time, but that it is controlled and regularly monitored throughout the year covered.

Table 5.1 Extract from an expenditure cash flow budget control sheet: year to 30 June 2000

	Annual budget (£)	July 1999 Actual (£)	August 1999 Actual (£)	Year to date (£)
Drugs and appliances	2000	–	100	100
Locum fees	3000	–	–	–
Relief service fees	1000	50	50	100
Hire and maintenance of equipment	1500	200	150	350
NHS levies	500	–	–	–
Training costs	600	50	30	80
Books and journals	100	–	20	20
Staff salaries (inc. PAYE/NIC)	30 000	2500	2350	4850
Registrars' salaries (inc. PAYE/NIC)	15 000	1250	1250	2500
Staff welfare	1000	100	50	150
Recruitment costs	500	–	80	80
Rates, water and refuse	5300	400	400	800
Light and heat	1500	–	150	150
Repairs and renewals	2000	500	100	600
Insurance premiums	800	–	200	200
Cleaning and laundry	2000	200	200	400
Garden maintenance	500	50	20	70
Printing, postage and stationery	1800	500	200	700
Telephone	4800	500	200	700
Accountancy fees	4200	–	–	–
Bank charges	200	–	100	100
Professional fees	200	–	100	100
Sundry expenses	1500	200	100	300
TOTAL BUDGETED COSTS	80 000	6500	5850	12 350

There is absolutely no point in having a budget if this is then filed away and forgotten about, or if all parties are not committed to achieving the budget.

There will always be unforeseen items which cannot reasonably be taken into account at the time the budget is prepared, and some practices choose to include a contingency fund to cater for such items. There may be unforeseen repairs required to the building; a partner may be required to take sickness or maternity leave which involves the partnership in additional locum expenses; there may be exceptional increases in telephone, cleaning and heating charges. Where such a contingency is operated, however, it should be treated as precisely that and the facility not abused.

It is essential to maintaining control that the budget is reviewed at regular (no more than monthly) intervals, and the partners should be made aware of any exceptional variances.

It should go without saying that such a budget cannot be efficiently formulated or monitored without an efficient and up-to-date book keeping system, which is considered in more detail in Chapter 8.

Let us now consider some of the areas where expenditure can be moderated and which are always worth looking at.

Locum fees

Are these really necessary? Locums are expensive and should only be engaged very much as a last resort. If it becomes necessary to engage locums on a regular basis, then the practice may be well advised to consider the recruitment of an additional partner, an assistant, an associate, or a retainer, for whom allowance might be claimed. These options are obviously subject to the practice meeting various criteria set out in The Red Book.

Relief service fees

Again, many practices consider these necessary, but they too are expensive and, particularly with small practices or those with low list sizes, the doctors should really ask themselves whether they can be afforded.

Telephone charges

Explore means by which telephone costs might be reduced; there are many schemes available from all telephone provider companies, which offer reduced charges. It is also worth shopping around between suppliers for better deals.

Do not wait for long periods for people to come to the telephone. Ask them to ring you back and they will then pay for the call.

Printing and stationery

Try to have the practice printing done at regular intervals and in bulk. Huge savings can be obtained here.

Open an account with a local stationer, or with one of the direct suppliers, where large discounts are frequently available.

Again, shop around. There are numerous stationery suppliers who will desire your custom, and don't be afraid to ask for a discount.

Postage

Explore the use of a lockable franking machine; keep a minimum of stamps available in the surgery – they are a constant temptation for people wishing to post their private mail. Avoid keeping loose stamps available in the surgery over Christmas.

Accountancy fees

Agree a fixed fee for preparation of the partnership accounts, partnership Tax Return and partners' personal tax affairs. Consider a monthly standing order arrangement to avoid the one-off large bill. Try to avoid firms who use hourly charging rates, as large bills can accumulate very quickly. If additional work is necessary over and above the standard compliance work, negotiate a fixed fee for that work also.

It is difficult to be specific as conditions vary from practice to practice and from region to region, but as a general rule of thumb a single-handed practitioner might be likely to pay a fixed annual fee of £1500 plus VAT, a five-partner practice might expect to pay £1000 plus VAT per partner, and a ten-partner practice perhaps £800 plus VAT per partner. These are the level of charges for employing specialist medical accountants who can provide a wide range of advice to the practice and individual partners.

Bank charges and interest

Above all, try not to go overdrawn, particularly with unauthorised overdrafts. Banks will charge a draconian rate of interest and a set penalty for each day that this overdraft continues.

Generally shop around and try to find the lowest overall rates. If you feel that the bank has been overcharging you constantly, there are organisations now in business who will examine bank charges and in a few cases substantial amounts have been recovered.

By and large, however, if you fail to treat a bank properly you will find it expensive. In particular, the use of cash flow forecasts (*see* Chapter 6) can be hugely beneficial in ensuring that unexpected overdrafts do not arise.

Remember, above all, that bank managers have extreme discretion over charges made to their customers' accounts. A GP partnership – particularly a large partnership where the annual turnover may well exceed £1m – is extremely lucrative business for a banker and huge dividends could well result from a visit to the manager to discuss charges on a general basis.

Again, be prepared to negotiate, and consider moving the property mortgage to the new banker as an added incentive to the bank manager, but be aware of early redemption penalties on your existing mortgage, or other conditions of the existing or new mortgage.

Summary

- Overall, do not be afraid to negotiate. Most suppliers expect it, and if you do not ask, you do not get. Shop around, and play one supplier off against another to get reduced prices.
- Agree fixed fees where possible and pay by monthly standing order, or direct debit (provided additional charges are not levied for this service) to improve cash flow.
- Really consider whether a cost represents value for money, or if it is truly necessary. Ask yourself, what are the alternatives.

6 Cash flow: problems and principles

Most businesses are able to maintain an acceptable and regular cash flow through the systematic issue of invoices and statements, together with an efficient system of credit control.

Few of the problems generally associated with this system affect the typical practice, where most income is received on a regular basis, with monthly and quarterly remittances from the HA. It is with regard to outgoings from the practice account and, in particular, drawings by individual partners that control of cash flow is most important.

The cash flow forecast

While a historical record of cash passing through the practice is essential, the systematic production of cash flow forecasts for up to a year hence is equally beneficial. These should look at the manner in which income will be received and outgoings paid, from which it will be possible to control the balance in the bank account on any given date, together with achievement of the budget (*see* Chapter 5).

It should be emphasised that such a forecast is not a projection of profit, but merely of the movements of cash, which for this purpose includes the practice bank accounts. Opinions vary as to exactly how long a period such a forecast should cover, but it is usually taken that it will cover each accounting year; thus if a practice makes up its accounts to 30 June annually, then during May or June 1999 it should be considering the preparation of a cash flow forecast for the year to 30 June 2000. Alternatively, some cash flow forecasts are prepared on a 'rolling basis' such that when one month has been completed and actual figures obtained, a further month is added to the end of the cash flow. In this way, there are always 12 months of cash flow projected.

Preparation of a cash flow forecast is not necessarily as difficult as it sounds, particularly for a practice that has had an established system over many years, and whose bookkeeping system is such that the required information can be produced with a minimum of delay. It is, of course, essential that such a forecast is reviewed on a regular basis. This should be done at least quarterly, but preferably monthly. Many practices now present cash flow forecasts on spreadsheets included in computer programs. Those familiar with the Excel series of programs will find little difficulty in setting up and running such a system. Where this is done, amendments can be made easily, avoiding the need for complex mathematical calculations.

A practice may make a good profit and the financial accounts may apparently show a healthy financial position, yet it may still have cash flow problems. This will probably be due to the slow receipt of items of income or excessive drawings by the partners. This will only come to light through the completion of a cash flow forecast, which not only shows how much cash will be received, but when it is expected to be received and paid out.

Once prepared, such a forecast may be used for the planning of major expenditure or as a basis for a presentation to lending institutions in support of applications for loans or mortgages. It also facilitates the preparation of partners' drawings calculations, enabling these to be dealt with in a far more logical and realistic manner than might otherwise be possible. The control of balances held on the bank account can prevent unnecessary overdrafts and hence result in a significant saving in bank interest charges (*see also* Chapter 5).

Preparation of the cash flow forecast

To construct a cash flow forecast, perhaps the best starting point is the previous year's cashbook. This will provide a good indicator of major cash inflows and outflows (receipts and payments).

The level of detail used, i.e. the number of categories of inflows and outflows, can be varied, but it is recommended to use the same categories as for the practice budget. This then enables the budget to be broken down on a monthly basis, which in turn assists with control of that budget. In this way the totals for the budget should tie in with totals for the year in the cash flow forecast.

Beginning with the first month on the cash flow forecast review, for each category, using information from the previous year, as well as known fluctuations for the current year (e.g. increases in fees and allowances, notional rent review, new or retired partners etc.), decide on a realistic basis, the amount likely to be received or paid in the current month. Continue with each category and each month until 12 months have been completed.

The receipts are added together each month to form the total inflows. Similarly, the payments form the total outflows. The total inflows less the total outflows is known as the net inflows (or net outflows), and is added to the bank balance for the end of the previous month to determine the bank balance for the end of the current month. This is done for each month in the cash flow forecast and will identify potential peaks and troughs in the practice bank balance. These peaks and troughs can then be levelled either by maximising income, minimising expenditure or adjusting partners' drawings.

Drawings

Systems of drawings are many and varied, and are outlined in more detail in Chapter 14. It is essential that a proper system of drawings be implemented and this is an integral part of a cash flow forecast. Some practices prefer to equalise payments to partners, primarily for their own convenience and ease of personal budgeting, whereas others will pay out on the basis of funds accumulated in the bank account at the end of each month or quarter.

Whichever of these, or other, systems is used, a properly managed system of cash flow forecasting, offers the partners a clear idea of how much they are likely to be able to draw month by month, or quarter by quarter.

Figure 6.1 shows a typical practice's cash-flow forecast for April to March, and predicts the opening and closing bank balances for each month. This particular forecast envisages large withdrawals by the partners during June, at the same time that substantial amounts are paid out in respect of rates which are not reimbursed until the following month. On this basis, a decision could be made to spread partners' drawings more evenly over the year, in an attempt to eliminate the need for a substantial overdraft from June to November.

Receipts	April	May	June	July	Aug	Sept	Oct	Nov	Dec	Jan	Feb	March	Total
NHS fees/allowances	9500	9500	11 365	9800	9800	13 652	9800	9800	12 653	10 000	10 000	13 652	129 522
Staff salaries reimbursements	438	1294	1066	1003	1070	1107	856	908	927	927	998	1080	11 674
Registrars' salaries reimbursements	640	640	640	720	720	720	720	845	845	845	845	845	9025
Rent and rates reimbursements	750	750	750	2975	750	750	750	750	750	750	750	750	11 225
Drugs reimbursements	–	–	–	192	–	–	70	190	1296	–	16	–	1764
Insurance exams	300	78	250	220	443	401	249	419	426	777	215	312	4090
Cremation fees	21	–	21	–	23	42	–	–	42	21	–	–	170
Appointments	208	208	208	208	208	208	208	208	208	208	208	208	2496
Sundry fees	62	42	163	–	–	315	27	63	–	412	–	–	1084
Total receipts	11 919	12 512	14 463	15 118	13 014	17 195	12 680	13 183	17 147	13 940	13 032	16 847	171 050

Figure 6.1 A sample cash flow forecast: (i) receipts

Payments	April	May	June	July	Aug	Sept	Oct	Nov	Dec	Jan	Feb	March	Total
Staff salaries (inc. PAYE/NIC)	617	1822	1502	1412	1507	1559	1206	1279	1305	1305	1406	1521	16 441
Registrars' salaries (inc. PAYE/NIC)	640	640	640	720	720	720	720	845	845	845	845	845	9025
Locum fees	432	512	245	–	315	645	315	545	215	150	450	215	4039
Relief service fees	70	35	–	70	75	40	62	52	120	–	–	75	599
Drugs and instruments	172	–	–	56	200	1300	–	20	–	–	42	23	1813
Rent and rates	750	750	3725	750	750	750	750	750	750	750	750	750	11 975
Repairs and renewals	72	–	84	12	160	–	–	51	20	–	–	61	460
Petty cash	100	100	100	100	100	100	100	100	100	200	100	100	1300
Loan interest	423	389	532	423	398	452	396	401	463	363	431	462	5133
Loan repayments	500	500	500	500	500	500	500	500	500	500	500	500	6000
Accountancy fees	–	1500	262	–	500	352	300	–	123	–	–	273	3310
Insurance	–	–	–	–	–	750	–	–	–	840	–	–	1590
Lighting and heating	–	98	–	55	46	–	–	62	59	–	–	–	320
Bank charges and interest	–	–	96	–	–	162	–	–	73	–	–	106	437
Telephone	–	–	839	–	–	433	–	–	926	–	–	519	2717
Drawings	7500	7500	12 636	7900	7900	7900	7900	7900	7900	7900	7900	7900	98 736
Sundries	72	–	735	42	78	24	924	–	–	2460	260	107	4702
Total payments	11 348	13 846	21 896	12 040	13 249	15 687	13 173	12 505	13 399	15 313	12 684	13 457	168 597
Net cash flow	571	–1334	–7433	3078	–235	1508	–493	678	3748	–1373	348	3390	2453
Opening bank balance	1604	2175	841	–6592	–3514	–3749	–2241	–2734	–2056	1692	319	667	1604
Closing bank balance	2175	841	–6592	–3514	–3749	–2241	–2734	–2056	1692	319	667	4057	4057

Figure 6.1 *cont'd.* A sample cash flow forecast: (ii) payments

7 Business planning for the general practice

It is amazing how many sizeable medical partnerships, which in many ways run as efficient businesses, nevertheless have no real plan for the future, operate without an efficient forecasting system and generally run on a day-to-day basis without any effective planning process.

For several years the Department of Trade and Industry (DTI) ran a business planning scheme, in which a high proportion of professional fees were paid by the DTI. This has now ended, although it is perhaps a salutary lesson that no more than 3% of general practices in the United Kingdom are understood to have taken advantage of it.

A GP who wished to save to take his family on a motoring holiday on the continent would become involved in all manner of forms of planning, almost certainly many months in advance. Ferries would have to be booked, routes planned, hotels arranged and the like. Almost certainly this would be done efficiently and the whole operation would run quite smoothly. Why, then would the same GP be reluctant to run his own business on a similar basis?

Some practices were obliged through their membership of the GP fundholding scheme to prepare business plans, but by and large these were confined to the fundholding facility and had little relevance to the business of the general practice.

This chapter looks at the manner in which business planning can take place, considers some of the options available and encourages practices to prepare their own plans on a regular basis.

What is a business plan?

By and large, a business plan represents a forward-looking, systematic approach to running a business, with which many GPs agree in theory but are reluctant to implement in practice. Only by looking ahead, and setting down in clear and concise terms the path it expects to follow in the next few years, can any business run in an entirely successful manner, whether it be a giant multinational corporation, a corner shop or a general practice.

Such a plan may lead to either a consolidation or a decision to change course. Reduced to its essentials, a business plan should set out to answer the following questions:

1 Where are we now?
2 Where do we propose to be in five years' time?
3 How are we going to achieve this?

In practice, a period of five years is normally considered applicable to plans of this nature, although this could be varied by agreement.

The plan should incorporate a number of features: cash-flow forecasts (*see* Chapter 6); expenditure budgets (*see* Chapter 5); maximisation of income (*see* Chapter 1); examination of performance by statistics (*see* Chapter 11); staffing levels; and several others.

Who should do the work?

Many practices resist the idea of introducing outside consultants, preferring to save the cost and do the work themselves. One must question whether this is a misguided policy: an outside consultant can offer a degree of detachment not always possible if the plan is prepared in-house; internal political factors can be kept at bay and, indeed, an independent mediator may at times be able to resolve them.

The consultant should be prepared to sit down, both separately and collectively, with all the partners, and look at their ambitions and aspirations, the type of medicine they wish to practice and the level of earnings they wish to enjoy, etc.

He or she should be both experienced and knowledgeable about the affairs of general practice, understand how GP finances work and, above all, be used to dealing with non-corporate businesses, particularly partnerships.

What should it contain?

The exact structure and contents of the plan are a matter for initial discussion between the consultant preparing the plan and the partners for whom it is intended. In the case of DTI plans for a large busy practice, it is virtually impossible to look at every aspect of the practice's function within the prescribed period of 15 days. It is therefore necessary to be selective and to highlight problems which are apparent; indeed, those which may have caused the partners to consider going through the planning process in the first place.

All plans should, however, contain:

- a mission statement
- a SWOT analysis
- an action plan
- profit projections and cash-flow forecasts
- current activity levels and targeting of achievements
- environmental issues, including the standard of the practice premises, administration, organisation and staffing matters.

Above all, the plan should contain precise guidance as to exactly how it will be implemented.

The mission statement

This briefly sets out the overall philosophy of the practice and the partners, as well as taking into account the wishes of the staff and patients. For example, a mission statement for a typical practice could read:

... to provide a high level of patient care, taking into account the practice's commitment to the National Health Service, whilst at the same time maintaining an acceptable level of income for the partners and staff.

We believe this can best be implemented within the context of a friendly and informal practice, in which patients have regular access to the doctor of their choice, that offers a range of quality services and maintains a high-quality practice team.

The SWOT analysis

An essential part of the plan is the discussion and establishment of the 'strengths', 'weaknesses', 'opportunities' and 'threats' applied to the practice. This involves exploring how strengths and opportunities could be benefited from, and how weaknesses and threats could be counteracted. Figure 7.1 shows a typical (but abbreviated) SWOT analysis for a sizeable practice.

Implementation and monitoring

The completed plan should set out the current situation and look at how proposed aims can be achieved over a five-year period. As a long-term plan, it should be flexible enough to incorporate changes that will inevitably be necessary in response to environmental or political factors.

It goes without saying that the plan should not be left to gather dust in a drawer, but should be monitored on a regular basis; the proposals, which

Strengths

- good premises
- high quality of young partners
- loyal and committed staff
- high level of activity in health promotion clinics
- large list sizes generate good capitation income
- commitment to the NHS
- practice fully computerised

Weaknesses

- difficulty in meeting targets
- low level of proceeds from night visits
- high expenditure on deputising
- branch surgery generating insufficient income
- senior partners of similar age
- difficulty in patient communication due to lower social class
- some partners not interested in expanding practice
- long waiting times annoy patients

Opportunities

- new housing estate being built
- additional marketing activity
- apply for additional partner
- formulate new rota to do more night visits
- utilise available space more efficiently
- introduce staff training scheme

Threats

- three senior partners likely to retire within next five years
- practice manager likely to move away within two years
- patients leaving through difficulty in obtaining appointments
- effect of national policy on GPs' income levels

Figure 7.1   A typical SWOT analysis

should have been accepted by the partners before the plan is finally formulated, should be implemented on the dates projected.

How to go about it?

Those GPs who feel they would benefit from the business planning process are strongly advised to appoint a consultant specialising in this field, who would initially meet the partners, draw up a plan of action and terms of reference, and set out details of likely costs.

It should then be possible for the practice to go ahead with the business plan to the benefit of all concerned.

What will it cost?

The short answer is that it need not cost very much at all. However, bearing in mind one of life's immutable truths, one largely gets what one is prepared to pay for.

One can indeed spend large amounts of money using outside consultants who may well, as indicated above, be able to take a more independent view than by having the plan prepared within the practice. This is a decision which only the partners can make.

A small crumb of comfort is that, however much it costs, this is a legitimate charge for taxation purposes against partnership profits and the partners will be likely to effectively receive tax relief at 40% on any such cost.

8 Basic book-keeping and accounts

General practice is big business: even a small practice has a turnover running well into six figures. Most conventional business enterprises of this scale employ skilled accounting staff, so the problem of inadequate records would not apply. Doctors, however, are notoriously bad at keeping records.

Most doctors have had no financial training. On entering general practice, however, they could become, within a relatively short period, equity partners in a medium-sized business enterprise. GPs then have to participate in decisions affecting: the finances of themselves, their partners and their staff; employment and staffing; budgeting and controls; taxation, insurance, banking and investment.

Financial decisions, which have to be taken regularly in all medical practices, are virtually impossible without access to well-maintained and comprehensive accounting records. Such records should be kept, or supervised, by a competent practice manager and they should form the basis of the practice's financial reporting facility, as sensible business decisions cannot be made without them.

The prime reasons for having book-keeping records are:

- to identify items of income and to highlight means by which this can be maximised
- to monitor expenditure and, through successful budgeting, control costs and economise (*see* Chapter 5)
- to draw up meaningful cash flow forecasts (*see* Chapter 6)
- by means of the above, to maximise profits and hence the earnings of the partners
- to comply with a clause in the partnership deed, which may specify that 'proper book-keeping records shall be kept'
- to enable the presentation of accurate information to the Inland Revenue
- to minimise accountancy fees
- to comply with the law. Since the introduction of Self-Assessment, it is a requirement to maintain up-to-date and accurate accounting records. Failure to do so could render the practice liable to Inland Revenue penalities.

Occasionally professional accounting firms keep the books of a practice, but this is likely to be expensive. It is uneconomic to have a professional person dealing with routine book-keeping records, as GPs have the facility to recover a proportion of the costs of employing practice staff, including clerical staff such as book-keepers. An accountant's fees are not recoverable, either wholly or partly, from the Health Authority, and they include a 17.5% VAT charge. However, most accountants will be happy to advise staff on methods of writing up the books, and if necessary teach them how to do so, including provision of training on computerised systems.

The types of book-keeping records that should be kept are discussed below.

The main cash book

The main cash book is the basis of the practice accounting system. Unlike the petty cash book, it records the receipts and payments of monies paid into and withdrawn from the practice bank account. This is *not*, therefore, the same thing as a ledger.

The vast majority of the transactions passing through the practice will go straight into the partnership bank account. Cheques will be received and banked and the majority of Health Authority income may arrive by direct credit; cheques will be drawn at regular intervals for running expenses, staff wages, partners' drawings, etc., direct debits and standing orders will pass through the bank account.

All of these should be recorded in the cash book, always up to date and maintained at regular intervals. Figure 8.1 shows a possible layout for an analysis cash book.

The member of staff responsible should aim to:

• balance the book periodically, at least monthly
• reconcile this balance regularly with the bank account statements.

Buying the book

There are a number of excellent analysis books on the market, e.g. the 'Guildhall' and 'Cathedral' systems and several other series offering a large variety of columns at each opening. Make sure you buy the right book; if in doubt, take along someone knowledgeable to advise you.

How many columns?

There should be sufficient columns of both receipts and payments to reflect adequately the transactions of the practice. This will, of course, vary according to the nature of the practice. For instance, in a large practice with a significant income from dispensing work, private patients or outside

Receipts

1997	Details	TOTAL	NHS	Appoint-ments	Insurance exams, etc.	Sundry fees	Other receipts
Jan 1	Balance b/forward	2,653 94					2653 94
	H Smith – fee	5 –				5 –	
	ABC Insurance Co	9 –			9 –		
	DEF Insurance Co	9 –			9 –		
3	GHI Insurance Co	9 –			9 –		
	JKL Insurance Co	9 50			9 50		
4	Income tax repaid	127 85					127 85
	County College	350 –		350 –			
5	MNO Insurance Co	9 50			9 50		
	Private Certificate	2 –				2 –	
7	BJ Funeral–Crem fee	16 50				16 50	
11	PQR Insurance Co	9 50			9 50		
	STU Insurance Co	9 –			9 –		
13	Loamshire County Council	15 –				15 –	
14	Mr Jones – fee	20 –				20 –	
	Mr Brown – fee	25 –				25 –	
	Mr Williams – fee	30 –				30 –	
17	XYZ Nursing Home	500 –		500 –			
	ABC Insurance Co	9 50			9 50		
18	DEF Insurance Co	9 –			9 –		
	Mr White	20 –				20 –	
	Loamshire FHSA						
20	Rent & Rates	2,350 –	2,350 –				
	GHI Insurance Co	9 50			9 50		
	Mrs Green	35 –				35 –	
22	Loamshire Hospital Clinical Assistant	108 96		108 96			
23	JKL Insurance Co	9 50			9 50		
24	Loamshire FHSA						
25	Trainee refund	3,647 94	3,647 94				
	JKL Insurance Co	9 50			9 50		
	ABC Insurance Co	9 50			9 50		
	Mr Black	56 –				56 –	
	Mr Blue	25 –				25 –	
28	Sundry cash takings	55 –				55 –	
	Cremation fee	16 50				16 50	
31	Loamshire FHSA						
	Monthly advance	7,250 –	7,250 –				
	Ancillary staff	1,300 –	1,300 –				
		£18,724 69	14,547 94	958 96	121 –	321 –	3781 79

Payments

1997	Details	Cheque no.	Sub no.	TOTAL	Salaries	Drugs & instru-ments	Registrar payments	Locum fees	Rent and rates	Lighting & heating	Cleaning	Tele-phone	Petty cash	Repairs & rentals	Partners drawings	Tax reserve transfers	Sundries
Jan 1	Dr Jones locum	635 46	1	100 –				100 –									
	Transfer	S.O.	1	1,200 –												1,200 –	
2	Building Society	47	2	85 76													85 76
	Fire Insurance	48	3	2,575 –													2,575 –
3	Accountancy fees	49	3	246 30			246 30										
	PAYE/NIC Month 9	49	4	896 40	651 10												
4	Smart Drug Company	50	5	35 65		35 65											
	Electricity Board	51	6	152 75						152 75							
	Mrs Jones cleaner	52		20 –							20 –						
	Petty cash	53		50 –									50 –				
6	Water Board	54	7	65 35					65 35								
9	Surgery rent	55	8	1,750 –					1,750 –								
	Gas Board	55	9	97 50						97 50							
11	Post Office Telephone	57		267 45								267 45					
	Mr Brown Plumb repair	58		25 –										25 –			
13	ZYX Instrument Co	59		15 50		15 50											
15	Dr Jones locum	60		150 –				150 –									
	Cleaning materials	61		27 50							27 50						
	Coffee	62		10 75													10 75
17	Legal charges	63		250 –													250 –
	Petty cash	64		50 –									50 –				
18	Mrs V Williams	64		266 45	266 45												
	Mrs J Smith	64		135 54	135 54												
20	Mrs B Jones	64		235 46	235 46												
22	Mrs D Johnson	65		226 92	226 92												
23	Mrs S Green	65		137 50	137 50												
	Mrs A Watson	7C		197 45	197 45												
24	Mrs M Robinson	7		226 45	226 45												
	Mrs L White	7		57 50							57 50						
25	Dr N Hunt trainee	7C		858 75			858 75										
	Borough Council & rates	S.O.		357 50					357 50								
	Staff pension scheme	S.O.		500 –													500 –
	Dr Grace	S.O.		2,200 –											2,200 –		
	Dr Hobbs	S.O.		2,000 –											2,000 –		
28	Dr Bradman	S.O.		1,950 –											1,950 –		
31	Dr Hutton	S.O.		675 –											675 –		
	Balance c/forward			868 56													
				17,856 13 £15,724 69	2,082 87	51 15	1,105 05	250 –	2,172 85	250 25	105 –	267 45	100 –	25 –	6,825 –	1,200 –	3,421 51

Figure 8.1 The GP's cash book: recommended column headings

appointments, the type and variety of income will be such that more columns will be required than in a more basic practice. Where necessary, advice should be sought on column headings.

All entries should be entered in a total column, as well as one of several analysis columns. Suggested column headings each side (receipts and payments) are listed in Boxes 8.1 and 8.2.

Box 8.1: The GP's cash book: recommended column headings – receipts

1 *Details*: all individual items of amounts paid to the bank in a single banking, e.g. 20 cheques of £20 each

2 *Totals*: e.g. £400 from details above, plus any direct credits by the HA or other bodies

3 *NHS fees and refunds*: all monies received from the Health Authority, e.g. monthly advances, quarterly cheques, rent, rates, ancillary staff and trainee repayments

4 *Outside appointments*: from schools, hospitals, nursing homes, etc., who pay regular fees to the practice. It may be helpful to keep a separate column for any fees taxed at source

5 *Insurance examinations*

6 *Sundry fees*: any payments which do not fall under the other headings. (Where justified by volume, it may be desirable to have a separate column for fees from private patients)

7 *Other*: e.g. tax repayments, transfers from other bank accounts, funds introduced by the partners, etc.

Box 8.2: The GP's cash book: recommended column headings – payments

1 *Cheque no.*

2 *Receipt no.*: the serial number of the receipted account for this particular payment. These should be numbered consecutively in a file maintained for that purpose (many practices choose to use cheque numbers for this purpose, eliminating the need for two numbering columns)

3 *Total*: all payments passed through your bank account, including those charged directly by the bank, e.g. bank charges and standing orders. Amounts entered into the total column should also go into one of several analysis columns (or into several columns where one cheque covers separate items)

Box 8.2: *continued*

Analysis columns

4 *Staff salaries*: payments to practice staff, *not* to partners or other doctors, or cleaners. Also enter amounts paid in respect of PAYE and NIC each month.

5 *Drugs and instruments*: for dispensing practices, payments to drug suppliers; otherwise all sundry payments for these items

6 *Registrar payments*: all net amounts, plus PAYE and NIC

7 *Locum fees*: including relief service payments

8 *Rent, rates and water*: all payments including those refunded by your Health Authority

9 *Lighting and heating*

10 *Cleaning*: payments to cleaners, their PAYE and NIC and purchase of cleaning materials

11 *Telephone*: surgery bills and partners' personal accounts, if relevant

12 *Repairs and renewals*: building repairs, plumbing and electrical work, repairs to equipment, etc., but *not* improvements or extensions or purchases of new equipment

13 *Partners' drawings*: either use one column for each partner or enter all partners' drawings in the same one (these are not salaries and should not be shown in the salaries column)

14 *Tax reserve transfers*: some practices operate a tax reserve system, by which transfers are made monthly to a building society account

15 *Sundries*: normally items which occur with insufficient frequency to justify a separate column, e.g. accountancy fees, bank charges/interest, purchase of new equipment, insurance premiums, etc.

Direct debits and credits

These comprise receipts that are paid directly into the practice bank account by a third party, and payments made by standing order or direct debit.

Direct credits may be advised to you by your HA or insurance company, and can be entered into the cash book at that time; otherwise they should be entered when they appear on your bank statement.

Where direct debits are known to be occurring monthly, an entry can be made in the cash book at the appropriate date; otherwise enter them when you receive a bank statement. All such items must be entered in the total column and the appropriate analysis column in the cash book.

Balancing the cash book

First check the mathematical accuracy of the entries you have made. Add up the total column and the various analysis columns, for both receipts and payments. It can be helpful to do this in pencil until you are satisfied that the figures are correct. A 'cross cast' can then be made, i.e. check that the total of all the analyses columns equals the total of the 'total' column (*see* Figure 8.1).

Then add the total receipts to the balance for the previous period, and deduct the total for payments. This gives the balance at the end of the current period. This is called a cash book summary (*see* below). Although this produces the true bank balance, it is unlikely that it will be identical to that shown on the bank statement: an explanation of why and how to reconcile the bank balance is given below.

Cash book summary

	£
Balance b/fwd at 1 October 1998	1763.40
Add: Receipts for month	29 930.55
	31 693.95
Less: Payments for month	13 410.04
Balance per cash book at 31 October 1998 b/fwd	18 283.91

Reconciling the bank

It is essential to check the cash book entries against the monthly bank statement, and to reconcile the balance shown. The steps to achieving this are given below.

1 Obtain the relevant bank statement(s).
2 Check the credit entries on the bank statement column, by comparing entries on the right-hand side with your receipts total in the cash book. Some entries in the cash book may not appear on the bank statement until the following month; these are called 'late credits'.
3 Check the payments (left-hand column) as above. Monies paid out, which do not appear on the current month's statement, are called 'unpresented cheques'.
4 Ascertain the balance carried forward per the cash book summary (*see* above).
5 Rule off the bank statement entries at the same date.
6 List the late credits.
7 List the unpresented cheques.

8 Write down the balance on the bank statement at the date the statement has been ruled off, and add to this the 'late credit' items to make a subtotal.

9 Subtract the total of the unpresented cheques from the subtotal.

If the balance obtained agrees with the balance according to the cash book summary, then the bank statement has been reconciled. If they do not, a repeat check should be made to identify the cause of the difference.

Bank reconciliation

		£	£
Balance per bank statement at			
31 October 1998			5369.38
Add: Late credits			15 000.00
			931.63
			462.50
			21 763.51
Less: Unpresented cheques	054668	262.50	
	054669	342.70	
	054670	191.00	
	054671	150.00	
	054672	981.30	
	054673	982.40	
	054674	569.70	
			3479.60
Balance per cash book at 31 October 1998			18 283.91

Box 8.3: Tips for writing up and balancing the cash book

- always keep up to date: it is easier to enter three or four cheques per day than all the month's cheques at once
- add up each page as you finish it (where possible finish a page at the end of a month)
- leave the top and bottom lines on each page vacant for the totals and brought forward figures
- be methodical: establish a routine that suits you and stick to it
- be consistent: always enter the regular items in the same column from month to month

---

Box 8.3: *continued*

- rule off at the year-end (say December 31) and leave two or three pages for late entries
- if your accountant takes the accounts away for a number of weeks at year-end, it may be advisable to use different books for alternate years; alternatively, use a loose-leaf cash book so that pages can be easily extracted
- enter on each cheque counterfoil the full details, e.g. 'Mr Brown: plumbing repairs: £5'
- zeros in the pence column confuse matters when adding up; use dashes instead
- always enter the date on the first entry of each day and show the year at the top of the page
- if, when checking against bank statements, items do not correspond, make inquiries with the bank immediately; if you delay, they may no longer have the information at hand
- do not attempt to reconcile the bank statement at longer periods than one month
- when reconciling a bank statement, *always* start with the bank balance and then adjust as indicated above

---

Manual cash books only provide limited information, and you will need to produce sub-analyses of each cash book column, to break down the practice earnings between categories included in the practice accounts. In some cases, it will also be necessary to analyse entries by doctor.

Due to the time-consuming nature of this, together with a propensity to errors, manual cash books are now used much less than was previously the case, with the majority of practices now using computer software for this function (*see* Chapter 10).

Salaries and wages

Full records of all calculations of staff salaries and wages must be kept. Where this is done 'in-house', entries are usually made in a ruled book showing:

- gross salary

- deductions for:
  - PAYE
  - Class 1 NIC (employees' contributions)
  - pension contributions (if applicable)
- net salary
- Statutory Sick Pay (SSP)/Statutory Maternity Pay (SMP) (if applicable)
- Class 1 NIC (employer's share).

The amount paid to the employee should correspond with the figure shown in the 'net salary' column.

Some practices calculate their salaries using a computer program such as Ferguson Payroll, which can be efficient and cheap. Several organisations now offer computerised payroll management for those practices without such facilities. Such companies can relieve the GP or practice manager of extra work and can make arrangements for direct bank transfers into the accounts of the employees concerned.

Computerised accounts

Some practices have chosen to adopt a book-keeping system based on a specialised computer program. GPs embarking on such systems should ensure that they suit the requirements of the particular practice and that they are designed to cater for the different demands of general practice.

Figure 8.2 shows suggested headings for a computerised cash book in a typical three-doctor practice.

DRS MORRIS, AUSTIN AND RILEY:
CASH BOOK COLUMN HEADINGS
Receipts
Main column heading   Subcolumn

FHSA quarter statement	Income	Practice allowances	
		Capitation fees	
		Registration fees	
		Item of service fees	Maternity fees
			Contraceptive fees
			Temporary residents
			INT & ET
			Vaccinations & immunisations
			Night visits
		Target payments	Childhood immunisation
			Pre-school booster
			Cervical cytology
		Sessional payments	Health promotion
			Minor surgery
		Seniority	Dr Morris
			Dr Austin
		PGEA	Dr Austin
			Dr Riley
		Leave advances received	Dr Morris
			Dr Austin
			Dr Riley
	Deduct	Superannuation	Dr Morris
			Dr Austin
			Dr Riley
		Superannuation: added years	Dr Austin
		Leave advances recovered	Dr Morris
			Dr Austin
			Dr Riley
		NHS levies	

Drugs refund
Rent & rates refunds
Ancillary staff refunds
Computer refunds
Hospital appointments
Other appointments
Insurance examinations
Cremations
Private patient fees
Sundry fees
Miscellaneous

Figure 8.2   Suggested cash book column headings: computerised accounts

Payments Main column heading	Subcolumn
Drugs and instruments	
Locum & relief service fees	
Hire and maintenance	
Practice replacements	
Medical subscriptions	
Medical books & journals	
Courses and conferences (Drs)	
Ancillary staff	Salaries
	PAYE/NIC
Staff expenses	Staff training expenses
	Recruitment costs
	Staff welfare
Rent & rates	
Insurance	
Lighting & heat	
Repairs & renewals	
Cleaning & laundry	
Postage & stationery	
Telephone	
Accountancy fees	
Bank charges & interest	
Capital expenditure	
Drawings	Dr Morris
	Dr Austin
	Dr Riley
Partners' tax	Dr Morris
	Dr Austin
	Dr Riley
Partners' NIC	Dr Morris
	Dr Austin
	Dr Riley
Loan repayments	
Petty cash	
Transfers to other a/c	
Sundries	

Figure 8.2 *continued*

9 Looking after the petty cash

All practices have cash passing through the surgery on a regular basis. First, one should consider what exactly is meant by petty cash. It literally means coins and bank notes, either received by the practice from patients as fee income or available in the form of a float, from which sundry cash disbursements can be made. These two aspects of petty cash in the average general practice should be kept entirely distinct.

The basic record for all cash transactions is the petty cash book, with the cash on hand on any given date being maintained in one or two petty cash boxes specifically used for that purpose.

The maintenance of an efficient and well-regulated system of petty cash recording is an integral part of the practice's book-keeping arrangements. While we may not be talking about large amounts of money, it does build up and, if it is not properly and efficiently recorded, can result in a great deal more trouble than it is worth.

Cash receipts

It cannot be emphasised too strongly that any fees received in cash, whether for certificates, cremations or sundry, should be properly accounted for and paid into the practice bank account without deduction.

The incorrect notion persists that these fees are in some way 'perks of office' which need not be accounted for and which the doctor is entitled to put into his pocket without paying tax. Nothing could be further from the truth; such fees are the income from his profession and it is essential that they are fully accounted for, both for accountancy and taxation purposes.

Cremation fees, for instance, have been traced by the Inspector of Taxes and doctors have been asked to pay tax on them, sometimes for several years in arrear. Such a liability, which may include interest and penalties as well as the tax loss, can amount to many times more than the tax 'saved' in the first place.

Cash receipts of this nature should always be collected and paid period-ically into the practice bank, at the same time as routine payments of cheques to the bank. Many practices retain cash in a special tin for a week or a fortnight, or until they reach an agreed sum, e.g. £50.

Much depends on the circumstances of the practice and the volume of fees received, but a policy should be established and strictly adhered to.

The petty cash book

It is strongly recommended that a separate book (*see* Figure 9.1) be kept to record the sundry fees received, not only as a routine record but also to

	SUNDRY CASH RECEIPTS - MAY 1998	Fees		Other		
May 1	Mr Brown – fee	2	50			
	Mr Smith – examination	5	85			
	Mrs Green – private patient	7	50			
2	Mr Jones – certificate		50			
	Staff telephone – refund			3	75	
	Mrs Harrison – private patient	5	25			
	XYZ Insurance Co – examination	7	00			
4	Dr Williams – locum fee	10	00			
	£	38	60	3	75	
	Paid to Bank 5/5/1998 £	42	35			

Figure 9.1   A specimen page from a sundry cash receipts book

enable the practice manager to check whether particular fees have been received.

The book should have a separate column for recording receipts of a non-fee nature and it is suggested that a separate column also be maintained for recording cremation fees.

Cash should be collected in a cash tin retained for this purpose only, which is cleared fully when the periodic bankings are made, as outlined above.

The mixing of sundry cash receipts of this nature with cash retained for payment of sundry petty cash items should be strongly discouraged.

Cash payments

A separate cheque should be drawn periodically from the bank for sundry small payments, based on an average weekly or monthly expenditure and replenished from time to time by a cashed cheque drawn on the practice bank account. This too should be kept in a separate cash tin maintained for payment purposes. Doctors and staff requiring cash for any purpose should be asked to complete a petty cash voucher or submit a receipt.

Once made, all such payments should be regularly and systematically recorded in a petty cash book used only for this purpose. This should ideally be in the form of an analysis book, which should be regularly added up, balanced and reconciled with the cash held in the tin. A specimen page from a typical payments petty cash book is shown in Figure 9.2.

Receipts, in the form of cash withdrawn from the bank, should be shown on the left-hand side. Payments should be shown on the right-hand side, being entered once in the payments (or 'total') column and again in the most appropriate analysis column.

The headings of the various analysis columns depend largely on the circumstances of the practice, but again they should be totalled periodically and, if the entries have been made correctly, the sum of the total of the various analysis columns should equal that of the payments column. These can all be totalled monthly and a balance carried forward to the start of the following month.

A test balance can be taken at any time, merely by finding the difference between the running totals of the receipts and payments columns. This should then be compared with the cash held in the tin and any difference investigated. Differences may well occur, usually for entirely innocent reasons, e.g. a payment might have been omitted from the petty cash book or an incorrect entry made.

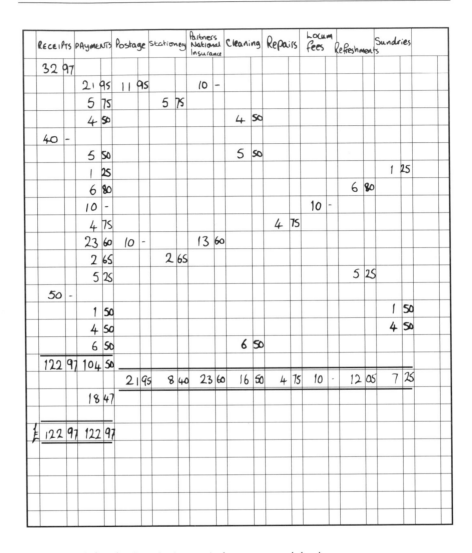

Receipts	Payments	Postage	Stationery	Partners National Insurance	Cleaning	Repairs	Locum Fees	Refreshments	Sundries
32 97									
	21 95	11 95		10 -					
	5 75		5 75						
	4 50				4 50				
40 -									
	5 50				5 50				
	1 25								1 25
	6 80							6 80	
	10 -						10 -		
	4 75					4 75			
	23 60	10 -		13 60					
	2 65		2 65						
	5 25							5 25	
50 -									
	1 50								1 50
	4 50								4 50
	6 50				6 50				
122 97	104 50								
		21 95	8 40	23 60	16 50	4 75	10 -	12 05	7 25
	18 47								
£ 122 97	122 97								

Figure 9.2 A few days' entries in a typical payments cash book

---

Box 9.1: Petty cash recording

Do:

- keep the cash proceeds from cash fees separate from cash used for making payments
- record cash fee income and pay into the practice bank account regularly
- make petty cash payments from a float withdrawn from the bank for that purpose
- record payments in an analysis cash book
- total the columns for each month and balance them
- reconcile the balance regularly with the cash held
- ensure that petty cash drawn from the bank is recorded identically in both the petty cash receipts book and the main cash book (*see* Chapter 8)

Don't:

- mix up proceeds for cash fees with sundry cash payments
- keep inadequate records
- fail to count the cash regularly and check the balance

Security

A few practices entirely eliminate the need to keep funds for payment of sundry cash items; it is certainly good policy to try and keep them at as low a level as possible. For instance: all staff wages/salaries should be paid either by bank giro credit or monthly cheque; postage stamps can be bought by cheque periodically from the post office; and classic petty cash items, such as milk deliveries, groceries and stationery, can all be converted to monthly accounts. If these are excluded, the need for substantial levels of cash in the surgery is very much reduced, enabling a far higher level of security.

10 Understanding practice accounts

All medical practices have a statement of accounts prepared on an annual basis so that the accounts are drawn up to a fixed accounting date each year. Most practices employ a specialist accountant to act for them in several different capacities. The duties the accountant should perform for the average medical practice are discussed in Chapter 32, but perhaps one of the accountants' main functions is the preparation of the annual accounts.

Some GPs question the need for accounts and feel that they are paying large amounts of money in professional fees for a document that they do not really need and which they may not fully understand. The purpose of this chapter is to examine the reasons why accounts should be drawn up and then to explain how they can be read and understood.

The major reasons why accounts are so necessary to the GP and his practice are listed in Box 10.1 and discussed in detail below.

1 *Tax*. Accounts are essential for agreeing the Self-Assessment tax liability of the individual partners. This equally applies in the case of a sole practitioner.

   If accounts cannot be produced, the GP, or his accountant, will be unable to determine the level of profits upon which tax liabilities are based, and he could find himself paying far more tax than necessary.

2 *Loan finance*. It is invariably necessary to present a set of accounts when approaching banks or other lending institutions to borrow money. This is the case irrespective of whether the money is for a surgery development project or for the personal use of an individual partner, such as for the purchase of a private house or car.

3 *Practice management*. A well drawn-up set of accounts, giving valuable information concerning the profitability and running of the practice, is essential when determining the success of the practice in financial terms; as a base for formulating future budgets and calculating drawings; and when taking decisions on the admission of new partners.

4 *Income sources*. Accounts drawn up on this basis may highlight additional means by which the practice can generate income, from both NHS and non-NHS sources. This is important bearing in mind the manner in which GPs' projected income is calculated, with emphasis on efficiency

and specified targets. It is therefore important to consider the level of income realised, as outlined in detail in Chapter 11.

5 *Cost economies.* A look at a logically drawn-up schedule of practice expenses for a year may help partners to identify means of cutting costs and hence increasing profits (*see* Chapter 5).

6 *Partnership deeds.* In a practice with a properly drawn-up partnership deed, there will be a clause requiring annual accounts to be drawn up, specifying the accounting year-end, that a professional firm of accountants will be used (and its name) and that the accounts must be signed by the partners as a true record.

7 *Capital and current accounts.* In many partnerships the allocation of these is complex (*see* Chapters 15 and 16) and it is essential that they be controlled in order to preserve fairness between the partners. Again, this is specified in many partnership deeds, but only by the production of regular and comprehensive annual accounts can control be effectively maintained.

8 *New partners.* Accounts can be an aid to recruiting suitable new partners, who may decline to join a practice which cannot produce a set of accounts from which they can ascertain their likely future earnings (*see* Chapter 13).

Box 10.1: Why do GPs need accounts?

- to agree practice tax liabilities
- in support of applications for loan finance
- as an essential management tool
- to highlight possible new income sources
- to make expenditure economies
- required by partnership deed
- for equity between partners
- to inform new partners
- to make appropriate arrangements when a partner leaves

Audited accounts

The word 'audit' is frequently used incorrectly and unadvisedly in referring to GPs' accounts. GPs and their partnerships, of whatever size, are not limited companies and there is no legal requirement to have an audit performed. Indeed, in many cases practices would consider it prohibitively expensive to do so. In this context, the term should be avoided at all costs.

Frequently, and particularly where accounts are required to be submitted in support of loan applications, a bank or building society will request the production of 'audited accounts'. They should be advised that the term is inapplicable and that the accounts are not audited. The fact that the accounts are not audited does not presume a lowering of standards and the GP should expect his accounts to be prepared to the highest possible professional standards.

The accountants who prepare the accounts should include on their certificate some form of wording to the effect that 'we have not carried out an audit', or similar.

Choice of year-end

Many practices have established year-ends and do not seek to change them. However, in some cases, particularly when new practices are being set up or a sole practitioner takes over from a retired doctor, there is an opportunity to decide a year-end for future use. It is suggested that several criteria be taken into consideration.

1 More accurate accounts, and hence more meaningful figures, tend to result from accounts prepared to a conventional quarter-end, i.e. 30 June, 30 September, 31 December and 31 March, because all NHS finances are organised on a quarterly basis. Where other year-ends are in force, it may be necessary to make apportionments and estimates which may not be entirely accurate.
2 For many years, it was conventional practice to prepare accounts to the earliest quarter-end within the accounting year, usually 30 June. However, a rather different agenda has now emerged with the introduction of the current-year basis of assessment. Whilst it may well not be advisable to change an existing year-end, where a new practice is being set up, or an opportunity otherwise arises, there may be great benefit in changing the year-end to 31 March. This is considered in rather more detail in the section on practice taxation (*see* Chapter 23).
3 Once a year-end is established, it may be changed if the taxpayer (and the partnership) wishes, but it is essential that knowledgeable professional advice is taken to ensure that there is no detriment in terms of tax payable.

How to read a set of accounts

Pages 66–81 show a typical set of partnership accounts for a six-doctor GP partnership. A statement of this type should ideally be prepared by the practice accountant each year, as soon as practicable after the accounting year-end. The accounts themselves are of a style frequently published and correspond to the style in publications issued by the Institute of Chartered Accountants. They also provide for all recommendations regarding the layout of accounts – chiefly concerning the 'grossing up' principle – in the Red Book.

Most accounts prepared for general practices, particularly large practices, are long and complex. Many GPs feel that their accounts are made unnecessarily complex. In fact, GPs' accounts are complex because the modern practice is complex, with its business activities spread over a number of separate functions. The partner should have greater cause for concern if his accounts did not fully reflect all the financial transactions of the practice over the year.

The accounts should be so designed as to take into account several aspects which are unique to general practice, and it is important that the following points are understood when reading the accounts.

1 *Comparative figures.* On pages 68 and 69, which set out the income and expenditure of the practice, it will be seen that the column on the right-hand side gives comparatives with the previous year's figures. These should always be shown in a set of accounts so that trends in income and expenditure are apparent. This also applies to the balance sheet on page 70 and the various supporting notes on pages 71–79.

2 *Profit for the year.* Page 68 shows that the partnership has realised a total profit for the year of £348 633, an increase of 7.5% on the figure of £324 229 shown for the previous year. It is important that the concept of profit is understood; this is the means by which businesses finance themselves and, in the case of general practice, from which the partners earn their respective income. NB. This is not the same as either salary or drawings (*see* 14 below).

3 *Income.* Page 69 sets out details of the income earned by the partnership during the year, through NHS fees, refunds and income from outside the NHS. Again, it is easy to obtain a comparison with the previous year.

4 *Payments.* Page 69 also shows the payments made by the practice during the year, and the manner in which the expenses have been divided, and further details are set out in the notes following.

5 *Profit-sharing.* Page 72 shows how the overall profits have been allocated between the partners.

In this case (Note 3) there were two changes in the partnership during the year. On 1 October 1998, Dr Orange, who previously had a share of the profits of 16%, achieved parity at 20%. On 31 January 1999, Dr Black retired and on the following day a new partner, Dr Grey, was introduced to the practice, with a 12% share of profits. As this is by no means uncommon in GP partnerships, it is important that the profits for the year are allocated between these separate periods in such a way that no partner loses out through this process.

6 *Separate profit-sharing periods.* For many years it was accepted practice to allocate profits on the basis of income and expenditure recorded in each separate profit-sharing period in force during a single year of account. This was both time-consuming and expensive, but was considered to be essential if an accurate allocation of profit was to be achieved. To a large degree, the situation changed with the advent of the 1990 GP contract, by which the incidence of practice allowances was greatly reduced. Thus the profits of a partnership became less dependent on the number of partners.

Since then, practices have invariably allocated profits on the time apportionment basis. This has avoided the additional cost of producing accounts on an 'actual' basis, and appears to be acceptable to GPs. The accounts of the sample practice, to which I refer, have been prepared in this manner. The lower part of Note 3 shows that the total profits for the year after deduction of prior shares (*see* 10 below) (£314 397) have been allocated on a monthly basis between the various profit-sharing periods in force. The profits shown in each of these individual periods have been allocated between the partners' profit-sharing ratios as applicable to each separate period.

It cannot be too strongly emphasised that a properly drawn-up set of accounts should show in some detail the manner in which profits are allocated between the various partners, including the distribution of prior shares of profit (*see* 10 below). Where applicable, rates of percentage or other method by which profits have been divided, should be clearly shown so that the partners are able to follow through the accounts the exact manner in which the profits have been divided and to see that the shares allocated to them are correct. Not only must equity be done, it must be seen to be done.

7 *The balance sheet.* This sets out, on page 70, the financial position as at any given date. It is normal practice for the accounts to be drawn up to the same date each year, in this case 30 June 1999. The balance sheet gives details of the assets and liabilities of the practice and, importantly, the manner in which the capital has been provided by the partners.

The partners' investment in the net equity of the surgery premises (property cost or valuation less outstanding mortgage) is shown in note 20 (page 78).

Similarly, the investment of the partners in the fixed assets and the working capital of the practice is represented by their capital accounts (Note 21, page 78), and the overall figure of £80 000 calculated as set out in Chapter 16.

This concept of capital in medical partnerships is complex, but it is necessary to understand it fully in order to understand GPs' partnership accounts. *See also* Chapter 23.

8 *Notes.* It is common for a number of items in the balance sheet and elsewhere to be set out in notes to the accounts – *see* page 71.

9 *Surgery ownership and income.* Note 16 (page 76) indicates that the practice owns its own surgery, which, in the balance sheet, is shown at a cost of £631 471. Further, the property capital accounts (Note 20), show that the surgery is owned by four out of the six partners: Drs Black, White, Green and Brown. Note 15 (page 76) specifies that the surplus on the property income and expenditure during the year (£2100) must be appropriated only to those four partners as joint owners.

Profits from this source are allocated between the four partners by crediting £525 to each of them (Note 2, page 71).

10 *Prior shares of profit.* Many practices have arrangements in force so that particular items of income are allocated between the partners in different ratios to the main practice profits. Note 2 refers to this principle as applying to: net surgery income; night visit fees; seniority awards; and the post-graduate education allowances. The partners have, in this case, agreed to retain their night visit fees, which have been allocated in the exact proportions in which they were earned; seniority and PGEA have been allocated on a similar basis, so that of the total profit realized (£348 633), a total of £34 236 is extracted before the remaining profits are allocated between the partners in agreed ratios.

11 *GP fundholding.* Although GP fundholding effectively ceased on 31 March 1999, for the year under discussion it was in force for part of the year and transactions affecting fundholding have therefore been passed through these accounts.

12 *'Grossing up'.* The details of income and expenditure (Notes 10 and 13) show that all expenses for which refunds are wholly or partially received (*see* Chapter 3) have been properly and fully grossed up. By this means, the accounts show the maximum level of expenditure in case of selection in the Review Body sampling process. This process has been applied in these accounts to: dispensing drugs; rates and water; staff salaries; registrars' salaries; and fundholding management allowance.

13 *Current accounts*. The partners' current accounts on page 80 are, in effect, their bank accounts with the practice. They give details of the profits earned by each partner and any additional credits, such as leave advances and income tax repayments, and details of payments, in terms of drawings, superannuation, national insurance, income tax, etc.

The final balances, provided that adequate funds have been set aside to provide for a working capital requirement, represent the undrawn profits of the partners, and can be withdrawn by the partners once the accounts have been approved and signed by all the partners. Failure to operate this equalisation procedure each year will almost certainly result in a 'snowball' effect, with the disparity between the partners' current account balances increasing steadily until it reaches an unacceptable level.

14 *Drawings*. Page 81 represents the cash withdrawals from the practice by the partners. Drawings are payments on account of the profits being earned by the partners (*see* Chapter 14). It is virtually impossible for these to be calculated accurately during the year, hence the need for the equalisation procedure outlined above. Nevertheless, it is helpful if a schedule of such drawings can be included in the accounts, so that the partners can check these figures against their own records.

15 *Dispensing*. The practice illustrated in the following pages is a dispensing practice and it will be seen that, for the information and guidance of the partners, a dispensing trading account (Note 23, page 79) has been provided.

In this illustration it will be seen that the profit on dispensing has increased dramatically over the year, from £5971 to £15 311, or a rise in the percentage rate from some 14% to some 41%. This may well have come about for a number of reasons, notably the facility to buy dispensing drugs at discounted prices.

It should be noted that in the main body of the accounts each of the figures should be shown on their proper side of the accounts in order to maintain the 'grossing-up' principle.

The practice manager should, in an enlightened and forward-looking practice, be made familiar with the practice accounts. In many partnerships, a separate set of the accounts are made available for her and she is expected to discuss them with the partners. The practice manager should also be invited to any meetings with the accountant.

It is normal for accounts, when completed and agreed by the partners, to be signed by them – a space in the accounts has been provided for these signatures on page 67. Signature of annual accounts is normally provided for in partnership deeds.

DRS BLACK, WHITE, GREEN, BROWN, ORANGE AND GREY
PARTNERSHIP ACCOUNTS
YEAR ENDED 30 JUNE 1999

Contents

Note The above page references are to pages in this book. In practice, pages 89 and 139 would be included within the statement of accounts, but are shown separately here for information purposes only.

DRS BLACK, WHITE, GREEN, BROWN, ORANGE AND GREY
ACCOUNTANTS' REPORT
YEAR ENDED 30 JUNE 1999

We have prepared the accounts for the year ended 30 June 1999 on records produced to us and from information and explanations given to us.

We have not carried out an audit.

TICK, FIDDLE & POST
Chartered Accountants

BRANCASTER
25 September 1999

CONFIRMATION BY THE PARTNERS

We approve these accounts and confirm that the accounting records produced, together with information and explanations supplied to Tick, Fiddle & Post, constitute a true and correct record of all the transactions of this practice for the year ended 30 June 1999.

....
Dr J W T Black

....
Dr D M White

....
Dr W J Green

....
Dr S J Brown

....
Dr M Orange

....
Dr A C Grey

DRS BLACK, WHITE, GREEN, BROWN, ORANGE AND GREY
DISTRIBUTION OF PROFIT
YEAR ENDED 30 JUNE 1999

	Page		1999 £	1998 £
Income	69		618 175	518 121
Expenditure	69		270 788	194 739
			347 387	323 382
Investment income	69		1246	847
Net profit			348 633	324 229

Allocated as follows:

	Prior shares (Note 2) £	Share of balance (Note 3) £	1999 Total £	1998 Total £
Dr Black	6279	37 466	43 745	69 752
Dr White	9374	66 286	75 660	71 946
Dr Green	6524	66 286	72 810	68 347
Dr Brown	5597	66 286	71 883	67 246
Dr Orange	5187	62 354	67 541	46 938
Dr Grey	1275	15 719	16 994	–
	34 236	314 397	348 633	324 229

DRS BLACK, WHITE, GREEN, BROWN, ORANGE AND GREY
INCOME AND EXPENDITURE ACCOUNT
YEAR ENDED 30 JUNE 1999

	Notes	1999 £	£	1998 £	£
Income:					
National Health Service fees	4	317 380		299 925	
Dispensing fees	9	3462		2546	
Reimbursements	10	191 960		182 797	
Appointments	11	61 466		19 428	
Other fees	12	12 478		13 425	
Fundholding management allowance	14	31 429		–	
Total income			618 175		518 121
Expenditure:					
Practice expenses	13	44 695		47 877	
Premises expenses	13	17 447		12 762	
Staff expenses	13	123 462		73 422	
Administration expenses	13	8270		7254	
Financial expenses	13	41 539		51 077	
Depreciation	17	3946		2347	
Fundholding expenses	14	31 429		–	
Total expenditure			270 788		194 739
			347 387		323 382
Investment income:					
Building society interest			1246		847
Net profit for the year (page 68)			348 633		324 229

DRS BLACK, WHITE, GREEN, BROWN, ORANGE AND GREY
BALANCE SHEET
YEAR ENDED 30 JUNE 1999

	Notes	1999 £	1999 £	1998 £	1998 £
Employment of funds:					
Surgery premises	16		631 471		627 524
Fixed assets	17		59 264		48 925
Current assets:					
Stock of drugs		4275		3940	
Debtors		12 946		13 869	
Balance at building society		6492		9421	
Cash at bank and in hand		12 465		232	
		36 178		27 462	
Current liabilities:					
Bank overdraft		–		3450	
Creditors		8642		7828	
Due to former partner	19	948		745	
		9590		12 023	
Net current assets			26 588		15 439
Net assets			717 323		691 888
Long-term liabilities:					
Property mortage	18		429 246		428 354
Net assets			288 077		263 534
Represented by:					
Partners' funds and reserves:					
Property capital accounts	20		202 225		199 170
Capital accounts	21		80 000		60 000
Current accounts	22		5852		4364
			288 077		263 534

DRS BLACK, WHITE, GREEN, BROWN, ORANGE AND GREY
NOTES TO THE ACCOUNTS
YEAR ENDED 30 JUNE 1999

1 Accounting policies

1.1 The income and expenditure account is prepared so as to reflect actual income earned, and expenditure incurred, during the year.

1.2 The stock of drugs is valued at the lower of cost or net realisable value.

1.3 Fixed assets are written off over their estimated useful lives. The following rates of depreciation are applied to the assets in use at the balance sheet date:

Furniture and fittings	– 10% per annum
Computer equipment	– 33⅓% per annum
Office and medical equipment	– 20% per annum

The surgery premises are not depreciated.

1.4 The income and expenditure for the year has been allocated between the periods shown in Note 3 on the time apportionment basis.

1.5 The accounts are prepared taking into account principles outlined in the General Medical Services Statement of Fees and Allowances.

2 Prior shares of profit

	Night visit fees	Seniority	PGEA	Net surgery income (Note 15)	Total
	£	£	£	£	£
Dr Black	1948	2625	1181	525	6279
Dr White	2264	4541	2044	525	9374
Dr Green	1846	2109	2044	525	6524
Dr Brown	2624	404	2044	525	5597
Dr Orange	3143	–	2044	–	5187
Dr Grey	412	–	863	–	1275
	12 237	9679	10 220	2100	34 236

DRS BLACK, WHITE, GREEN, BROWN, ORANGE AND GREY
NOTES TO THE ACCOUNTS (continued)
YEAR ENDED 30 JUNE 1999

3 Distribution of profit

	Period to 30 Sept 1998 %	Period to 31 Jan 1999 %	Period to 30 June 1999 %
Dr Black	21	20	–
Dr White	21	20	22
Dr Green	21	20	22
Dr Brown	21	20	22
Dr Orange	16	20	22
Dr Grey	–	–	12
	100	100	100

Share of balance:				Total
	£	£	£	£
Dr Black	16 506	20 960	–	37 466
Dr White	16 506	20 960	28 820	66 286
Dr Green	16 506	20 960	28 820	66 286
Dr Brown	16 506	20 960	28 820	66 286
Dr Orange	12 575	20 959	28 820	62 354
Dr Grey	–	–	15 719	15 719
	78 599	104 799	130 999	314 397

4 National Health Service fees

	Note	1999 £	1998 £
Allowances	5	61 060	59 262
Capitation	6	193 602	182 015
Sessional	7	16 691	18 250
Item of service	8	46 027	40 398
		317 380	299 925

5 Allowances

Practice allowances	32 220	30 802
Seniority awards	9670	9200
Post-graduate education allowances	10 220	10 625
Rural practice payments	4670	4395
Registrar supervision grant	4280	4240
	61 060	59 262

DRS BLACK, WHITE, GREEN, BROWN, ORANGE AND GREY
NOTES TO THE ACCOUNTS (continued)
YEAR ENDED 30 JUNE 1999

6 Capitation payments

	1999 £	1998 £
Capitation fees	143 400	137 664
Registration fees	8700	8500
Child health surveillance fees	6250	5938
Deprivation payments	4600	4200
Target payments:		
Cervical cytology	7850	6305
Childhood immunisations	9462	7462
Pre-school boosters	13 340	11 946
	193 602	182 015

7 Sessional payments

Health promotion payments	12 145	13 008
Asthma management	900	1390
Diabetes management	900	1390
Minor surgery	2746	2462
	16 691	18 250

8 Item of service fees

Night visits	12 237	9862
Temporary residents	6162	7871
Contraceptive services	8700	5879
Emergency treatment and INT	191	284
Maternity	12 619	10 716
Vaccinations and immunisations	6118	5786
	46 027	40 398

9 Other NHS income

Dispensing fees	3462	2546

DRS BLACK, WHITE, GREEN, BROWN, ORANGE AND GREY
NOTES TO THE ACCOUNTS (continued)
YEAR ENDED 30 JUNE 1999

10 Reimbursements

	1999 £	1998 £
Premises:		
Notional rent	42 364	42 364
Rates and water rates	10 465	8462
Staff costs:		
Salaries	60 610	35 209
Training	1346	–
Registrars' salaries	24 680	21 240
Computer maintenance	2750	1645
Drugs	49 745	38 877
	191 960	147 797

11 Appointments

Hospitals:		
Brancaster General Hospital (Dr White)	9648	8462
St John's Hospital (Dr Brown)	2645	2520
Other appointments:		
Police surgeon's fees	41 275	3246
Midworth Nursing Home	4275	3445
ABC Ltd	739	–
XYZ Ltd	1194	1755
St Peter's School	1690	–
	61 466	19 428

12 Other fees

Private patients	5249	5270
Insurance examinations etc.	5946	4280
Cremations	150	120
Sundry	1133	3755
	12 478	13 425

DRS BLACK, WHITE, GREEN, BROWN, ORANGE AND GREY
NOTES TO THE ACCOUNTS (continued)
YEAR ENDED 30 JUNE 1999

13 Expenditure

	1999 £	1998 £
Practice expenses:		
Drugs and instruments	37 426	35 462
Locum fees	421	3546
Relief services fees	3022	6084
Hire and maintenance of equipment	1275	843
NHS levies	462	420
Practice replacements	694	527
Medical books	750	575
Courses and conferences	645	420
	44 695	47 877
Premises expenses:		
Rates and water rates	10 465	8462
Heat and light	3469	2570
Insurance	1240	947
Maintenance and repair	1847	509
Cleaning and laundry	426	274
	17 447	12 762
Staff expenses:		
Salaries	89 132	44 901
Registrars' salaries	24 697	21 246
Training expenses	3962	1750
Recruitment costs	425	875
Staff welfare	5246	4650
	123 462	73 422
Administration expenses:		
Postage and stationery	408	925
Telephone	2546	2296
Accountancy fees	4390	3625
Sundries	426	408
Professional fees	500	–
	8270	7254
Finance expenses:		
Bank interest and charges	1275	2380
Property mortgage interest	40 264	48 697
	41 539	51 077

14 Fundholding management allowance

		1999 £	1998 £
Allowance received for capital expenditure	3071		
Allowance received for revenue expenditure	31 429		
		34 500	
Capital expenditure:			
Chairs	1150		
Carpets	1921	(3071)	
		31 429	
Revenue expenditure:			
Salaries	24 978		
Telephone	1346		
Stationery	924		
Training	1536		
Computer maintenance	1370		
Accountancy	1175		
Recruitment	100	31 429	
Net income		–	

15 Net surgery income (expenses)

	1999	1998
Notional rent	42 364	42 364
Property mortgage interest	(40 264)	(48 697)
	2100	(6333)

16 Surgery premises

	1999	1998
Freehold property:		
The Medical Centre, High Street, Brancaster		
At 1 July 1998	627 524	627 524
Additions during year	3947	–
At 30 June 1999	631 471	627 524

DRS BLACK, WHITE, GREEN, BROWN, ORANGE AND GREY
NOTES TO THE ACCOUNTS (continued)
YEAR ENDED 30 JUNE 1999

17 Fixed assets

	Furniture & fittings £	Computer equipment £	Office & medical equipment £	Total £
Cost				
At 1 July 1998	39 178	22 496	5283	66 957
Additions during year	3724	25 934	665	30 323
Less: FHSA grants	–	(12 967)	–	(12 967)
Fundholding management allowance	(3071)	–	–	(3071)
At 30 June 1999	39 831	35 463	5948	81 242
Depreciation				
At 1 July 1998	6425	10 962	645	18 032
Charge for year	1875	1562	509	3946
At 30 June 1999	8300	12 524	1154	21 978
Net book amounts				
At 30 June 1999	31 531	22 939	4794	59 264
At 30 June 1998	32 753	11 534	4638	48 925

18 Property mortgage

The practice has a mortgage loan with Branshire Bank plc, secured on the freehold property and repayable by monthly instalments over 20 years.

The term of the mortgage remaining is 16 years, the interest rate is variable at 1.25% over base and at 30 June 1999 was 8%.

The monthly repayments at present are £4275 and the capital outstanding is as follows.

	1999 £	1998 £
Balance at 30 June 1998	428 354	436 618
Net advances (repayments) during year	892	(8264)
	429 246	428 354

DRS BLACK, WHITE, GREEN, BROWN, ORANGE AND GREY
NOTES TO THE ACCOUNTS (continued)
YEAR ENDED 30 JUNE 1999

19 Former partners' accounts

	Dr H W Blue £	Dr J W T Black £
At 1 July 1998	745	
Less: Withdrawn	745	
	‗‗‗	
Transfer from partners' current accounts (page 80)		948

20 Property capital accounts

	1999 £	1998 £
Dr Black	50 557	49 793
Dr White	50 556	49 793
Dr Green	50 556	49 792
Dr Brown	50 556	49 792
	202 225	199 170
Represented as follows:		
Surgery premises (Note 16)	631 471	627 524
Less: Property mortgage (Note 18)	429 246	428 354
	202 225	199 170

21 Capital accounts

	1999	1998
Dr Black	–	12 600
Dr White	17 600	12 600
Dr Green	17 600	12 600
Dr Brown	17 600	12 600
Dr Orange	17 600	9600
Dr Grey	9600	–
	80 000	60 000

DRS BLACK, WHITE, GREEN, BROWN, ORANGE AND GREY
NOTES TO THE ACCOUNTS (continued)
YEAR ENDED 30 JUNE 1999

	1999 £	1998 £
22 Current accounts (page 80)		.
Dr Black	–	(927)
Dr White	2091	1276
Dr Green	1233	1705
Dr Brown	1648	1466
Dr Orange	1346	844
Dr Grey	(466)	–
	5852	4364
23 Dispensing Trading Account		
Dispensing fees	3462	2546
Drug refunds	49 275	38 887
	52 737	41 433
Cost of drugs dispensed	37 426	35 462
Profit for year	15 311	5971
Return	40.9%	14.4%

DRS BLACK, WHITE, GREEN, BROWN, ORANGE AND GREY
PARTNERS' CURRENT ACCOUNTS   YEAR ENDED 30 JUNE 1999

	Total £	Total £	Dr Black £	Dr Black £	Dr White £	Dr White £	Dr Green £	Dr Green £	Dr Brown £	Dr Brown £	Dr Orange £	Dr Orange £	Dr Grey £	Dr Grey £
At 1 July 1998		4364		(927)		1276		1705		1466		344		–
Profit for the year (page 68)	348 633		43 745		75 660		72 810		71 883		67 541		16 994	
Leave advances received	6625		–		1325		1325		1325		1325		1325	
Income tax repayment: 1995/96	5668		2746		1327		842		753		–		–	
Cash introduced	9000		–		–		–		–		–		9000	
	369 926		46 491		78 312		74 977		73 961		68 866			27 319
		374 290		45 564		79 588		76 682		75 427		69 710		
Less:														
Partners' monthly drawings (page 81)	260 029		41 523		53 139		52 558		48 027		51 228		13 554	
Superannuation:														
Standard	12 568		1466		2564		2564		2564		2193		1217	
Added years	7765		–		–		3529		4236		–		–	
Appointments	738		–		579		–		159		–		–	
Leave advances repaid	6445		958		1289		1289		1289		1289		331	
Income tax paid:														
1997/98	128		–		–		–		–		128		–	
1998/99	49 634		12 345		9387		9465		10 227		5246		2964	
PAYE deducted at source	4623		–		3628		–		995		–		–	
National Insurance: Class 1	1106		–		868		–		238		–		–	
Class 2	1399		160		280		280		280		280		119	
	344 435		56 452		71 734		69 685		68 015		60 364		18 185	
		29 855		(10 888)		7854		6997		7412		9346		9134
Transfers from property capital accounts (Note 20)	(3055)		(764)		(763)		(764)		(764)		–		–	
Transfers to capital accounts (Note 21)	(20 000)		12 600		(5000)		(5000)		(5000)		(8000)		(9600)	
Transfer to former partner's accounts (Note 19)	(948)		(948)		–		–		–		–		–	
		(24 003)		10 888		(5763)		(5764)		(5764)		(8000)		(9600)
Balances at 30 June 1999		5852		–		2091		1233		1648		1346		(466)

DRS BLACK, WHITE, GREEN, BROWN, ORANGE AND GREY
PARTNERS' MONTHLY DRAWINGS
YEAR ENDED 30 JUNE 1999

		Dr Black £	Dr White £	Dr Green £	Dr Brown £	Dr Orange £	Dr Grey £
	£						
1998 July		3000	3000	3000	3000	2300	–
August		3000	3000	3000	3000	2300	–
September		4352	3946	3564	3294	4784	–
October		3500	3500	3500	3500	2700	–
November		3500	3500	3500	3500	2700	–
December		5325	5125	4928	4265	5027	–
	(T)	2746	1327	842	753	–	–
1999 January		3500	3500	3500	3500	2700	–
	(C)	12 600	–	–	–	–	–
February		–	3500	3500	3500	3500	1700
March		–	6425	6274	5947	8247	3926
April		–	3800	3800	3800	3800	1800
May		–	3800	3800	3800	3800	1800
June		–	8716	9350	6168	9370	4328
	260 029	41 523	53 139	52 558	48 027	51 228	13 554

(C) Capital withdrawn
(T) Tax repayment withdrawn

11 Computerised accounts
Terry Taylor

Such has been the move towards information technology, that the majority of practices now choose to operate a computerised accounting system, such as the Maclean McNicholl GP Accounts Package.

There are many accounting systems available today, although not many are dedicated to GP finance. It is essential that you select a package which not only meets the demands of practice management to assist with maximising earnings, but also the requirements of the accountant, to minimise your accountancy fees. You should also consider your own technical (computer and accountancy) abilities, together with the suitability of your computer system.

Many specialist medical accountants also offer IT consultancy services and should be able to advise you on appropriate systems, as well as provide full training and support facilities. In addition, it is commonly possible to provide your accounting information to the accountant on a computer disk or by Email.

Some accountants profess to operate systems whereby accounting information is transferred automatically into their own accounting software. Whilst in principle this is a time-saving (and therefore cost-saving) idea, in practise, the accounting information must be rigidly maintained by the practice manager with little or no room for manoeuvre or variance in the practice circumstances. This can also be used as an excuse to charge additional accountancy fees on the basis that the accounting records have not been properly maintained, when in fact the problem is the rigidity of the accountants' software. This is not to say that such systems cannot work effectively, which they can, but often this is at a cost.

In purchasing accounting software the following need to be considered:

- Cost.
- Capabilities of the software.
- Ease of use.
- Flexibility.
- Capabilities of the user.
- System requirements.
- Support and training facilities.

- Practice management requirements.
- Accountants' requirements.

Cost

The cost of computerised accounting systems can vary wildly from less than £100 to several thousand pounds. Software costing thousands of pounds is generally aimed at accounting professionals and big businesses. These systems will often include many facilities that are superfluous to general practice.

Similarly, software that is at the very inexpensive end of the range may be aimed at home use and not include the necessary elements or flexibility that a practice requires.

An addition to the basic cost is often an annual maintenance and support charge.

Capabilities of the software

It is important that the software is capable of producing the correct level of information for the practice. For example, it will be necessary for the software to perform all of the functions of a manual accounting system (*see* Chapter 8).

In addition, some practices may require facilities to analyse data and produce charts and pictorials for reporting purposes.

There will undoubtedly be a few practices which employ technically skilled bookkeepers who may require facilities for including debtors and creditors and accounting to trial balance.

However, the most commonly required functions are listed below:

- Receipts and payments analysis.
- NHS analysis.
- Ability to cope with a number of bank, building society, loan and petty cash accounts.
- Facilities for inter-account transfers.
- Direct debit or standing order facilities.
- Able to cope with any accounting period.
- Bank reconciliation facilities.
- Printouts of data available.
- Backup capabilities.

Ease of use

There is little point in purchasing a computer package which is so difficult to use that the practice manager prefers the manual accounting system!

The best software is often menu driven, with each function available at the press of a single button, or click of a mouse. It is also helpful if similar functions throughout the software use similar keystrokes, as this facilitates memory by the user.

Systems with graphical images are also popular as this increases ease and pleasure of use.

Flexibility

Each practice and each firm of accountants acting for those practices will have slightly different preferences for the provision of information. For this reason it is essential that the software chosen can be adapted to the relevant needs of the user.

So what is meant by flexibility? It is important that the software provides a wide range of categories by which to analyse the receipts and payments. It is also necessary that these headings are relevant to the practice. But, in addition, the user must be able to add, delete, or change headings to fit in with their own practice. The system should be familiar with NHS receipts and payments, and the structure of Health Authority payments. It should also be possible to provide a wide range of printouts, some of which may be user definable, which clearly provide the information that has been input to the system. There is, after all, little point spending time entering detailed information, if that information is not usable.

Accounting software should also be capable of dealing with a wide range of types of transactions including direct debits, standing orders, transfers, petty cash entries, receipts or payments containing more than one category and so on.

Capabilities of the user

Not everyone is an accountant. Not everyone is comfortable with the use of high technology equipment. Not everyone is interested in becoming an accountant or computer whizz-kid. For these reasons, it is essential, if the practice is to make the most of their accounting software, that consideration is given to the ability of the bookkeeper.

Practices who choose the most detailed software with full accounting functions will be disappointed if the practice manager or other user of the program, has virtually never seen a cashbook before.

Therefore, the user should be involved in the decision-making process of choosing the software to ensure that he/she is comfortable with the system. This is the only way to ensure maximum efficiency both from the user and from the software.

System requirements

As with all software, the purchaser will come unstuck if the computer system is incapable of running the program. In actual fact, most accounting packages do not require vast computer resources to operate, although speed may be enhanced with a more powerful processor and higher memory. Many packages continue to be operable using DOS, although there is now a tendency towards Windows 95/98/NT. Generally speaking, Windows packages are faster to learn due to the graphical content and functions which operate throughout the packages. However, some people have a preference for the frequent simplicity of DOS programs.

Normally, a system using any Pentium processor (or equivalent) with 16 Mb RAM memory will be sufficient to operate accounting software. More detailed programs may require more power, whereas DOS software may still be capable of operating on a machine with a 286 processor and 1 Mb RAM memory.

Overall, check the system requirements with the supplier or your IT consultant.

Support and training facilities

It is advisable to buy only software where support and training facilities are available. This may be through your accountant, IT consultant or the software supplier.

Support is normally via a telephone hotline and should be able to answer any query you may have regarding the software.

Training is normally provided by a third party either contracted by the supplier or by the practice, e.g. the accountant.

Practice management requirements

Clearly, an accounting system will be of minimal benefit if it does not provide the information the practice needs. These requirements of the software need to be considered between the doctors, practice manager and accountant.

It is suggested that the following questions need to be answered:

- What will the primary purpose of the software be?
- Will the software be used to track receipts and payments fluctuations?
- Can NHS income be reviewed and analysed?
- Does the system provide comparisons with known averages?
- What analysis facilities does the package have?
- Does the package meet the requirements of all of the end users of the data?

The answers to these questions will almost certainly narrow down the choices available to the practice.

Accountants' requirements

If the practice selects a full accounting system with facilities to account to trial balance, then it is important that the user is capable of understanding and using *all* the facilities. A half-used full accounting system can be as bad as no accounting system at all.

If the practice selects what is essentially a computerised cashbook system, the accountant requires all accounts to be included on the system, with each transaction accurately analysed, but most importantly with the bank account(s) analysis reconciled to the bank statements.

It is these latter points which will serve to minimise the practice's accountancy fees.

Conclusion

There are many considerations in purchasing an accounting system, but the cost of the system will probably be saved in the first year accountancy fees if the correct system is chosen and used well.

Dean Taylor Associates provide a wide range of IT consultancy services, as well as traditional specialist medical accountancy advice.

For further assistance in choosing accounting software, please telephone: 01483 426711.

12 Financial statistics
Michael Gilbert

An advantage of medical practice, which is not readily available to other businesses, is access to statistics, which the GPs and their manager can use to judge the profitability and efficiency of the practice. Some of these statistics and their source are set out below.

Expenditure levels

By the averaging process, and for superannuation purposes, the DoH considers that the expenses of a medical practice currently run at about 34% of gross income. This is very low when one considers that this takes into account all items paid personally by the partners, including motoring and house expenses, and spouses' salaries, etc. It is to the GPs' advantage for taxation purposes that expenses be maximised, which can only be done by means of accounts drawn up in a manner that fully analyses the income and expenses of the practice. The Association of Independent Specialist Medical Accountants (AISMA) produces an annual survey of GP accounts covering a sample of approximately 15% of all GPs in the UK. So far as concerns expenditure for 1997/98, AISMA discloses the percentage expenses to total income of a medical practice as follows.

	%
Staff costs	27.3
Medical expenses	17.4
Premises	4.5
Administration	6.3
Finance	2.7
Depreciation	0.7
	58.9

AISMA also states that the average percentage staff reimbursement is 69.95%, which represents £12.68 per patient.

Income profile

The AISMA survey for 1997/98 breaks down the percentage total income of a medical practice as follows.

	%
	%
NHS fees and allowances	57.1
Reimbursements	39.5
Non-NHS income	8.8
	100.0

Proportions of NHS income

Figures currently available from the DoH suggest that the average proportions of NHS income received by a typical medical practice during 1997/98 would be as follows.

	%
Practice allowances	16.9
Capitation fees	52.2
Target payments	7.7
Sessional payments	5.6
Items of service fees	13.7
Other NHS income, including dispensing fees	3.9
	100.0

Average patient numbers

The NHS Executive produces figures giving average patient numbers per GP over the three age bands of the patients. They also provide information relating to the status of GPs in the UK, that is, how many are full time, part time, job sharers or three-quarter time. The number of patients per full-time equivalent GP can be calculated as follows, relating to 1998.

Age band	England	Wales	Scotland	Northern Ireland	Total UK
0–64	1677	1509	1343	1597	1629
65–74	169	171	136	133	162
75 and over	143	141	102	98	139
	1989	1821	1581	1828	1930

Item of service fees

The Health Departments annually provide averages of item of service fees earned by GPs on a per patient basis. This information is extremely valuable in attempting to evaluate the earnings of a practice. For 1997/98 the Returns per patient were as follows (United Kingdom):

Night visits	1.61
Maternity medical services	1.54
Contraceptive services	1.14
Vaccinations and immunisations	0.59
Temporary residents	0.37
Emergency treatment	0.08
	£1.33

Sessional payments

The Health Departments also annually provide averages of sessional payments earned by GPs on a per patient basis. For 1997/98 the figures are as follows (United Kingdom):

Health promotion	1.55
Minor surgery	0.62
	£2.17

Other income

Similar information to the above for 1997/98 is also available for other NHS income sources as follows (United Kingdom):

Child health surveillance fees	0.57
Registration fees	0.46
	£1.03

Total NHS income and expenses

It is possible to further evaluate the financial efficiency of a medical practice by comparing gross and net income levels, both on a partner and per patient basis. This is done by extracting figures from those published annually in respect of intended average remuneration levels by the Review Body on Doctors' and Dentists' Remuneration. These figures are available up to March 2000, although where year-ends other than March are used, they must be apportioned accordingly. The figures set out below show the UK averages for the three years to 31 March 2000.

	Year to 31 March		
	1998	1999	2000
	£	£	£
Intended average net remuneration	46 450	49 030	50 760
Add: Full-time equivalent basis	2555	2940 ⎫	
Higher target pay	3300	3500 ⎬	1840
	52 305	55 470	52 600
Less: Balancing adjustment	615	527	(432)
Expected average net remuneration	51 690	54 943	53 032
Expenses	23 200	23 400	24 700
Gross NHS fees and allowances delivered by way of the Pay Scale	£74 890	£78 343	£77 732

It is worth mentioning at this stage that to maintain a consistency of approach one should always translate the figures on to a full-time equivalent basis. Furthermore it is interesting to note that the Review Body expects GPs to earn the higher target pay which is built into the above figures, although the latest statistics available on target achievements reveal the following.

	Percentage of GPs achieving higher target pay
Childhood immunisations	85%
Pre-school boosters	83%
Cervical cytology	90%

Gross income, expenses and profit

By applying the income profile to the Review Body figures, it is possible to arrive at a profile which represents the gross income, expenses and profit of a typical full-time equivalent GP, which for 1997/98 was as follows.

Gross practice income per full-time partner	
– from NHS	74 890
– from other sources	11 736
	£86 626
Average expenses per full-time partner	
– relating to NHS	23 200
– relating to other sources	4045
	£27 245
Average profit per full-time partner	
– from NHS	51 690
– from other sources	7691
	£59 381

It is interesting to note that the level of expenses relating total non-NHS sources is 34.59%, which is similar to the figure set out under expenditure levels. This is less than the NHS expenses of 31% because non-NHS expenses do not attract reimbursement. The reality of the situation is that it is difficult to identify what the non-NHS expenses actually relate to, and one is led to the conclusion that the Review Body expense figure of £23 200 is short of what GPs are actually incurring. In this way, non-NHS profits will supplement NHS earnings to the amount of the expenses shortfall.

Based on the above, a national profile of a typical GP or practice can be built up, which is demonstrated in the following case study.

A case study

Reference to the accounts in Chapter 10 shows a set of typical GP partnership accounts which, although not bearing direct relation to any known practice, nevertheless gives statistics of the type GPs require to assess the financial performance of their practices, and subsequently to make management decisions and institute necessary economies. Figure 12.1 reproduces some statistics from these accounts.

The GP or practice manager interpreting these accounts has the following valuable items of information at his disposal.

• The practice has five constant, full-time equity partners, and the average patient list is 1912. Gross NHS income, both per partner and per

patient, is comfortably above the previous year's performance. However, gross NHS income is below the intended average due to the lower than average list size and the knock-on effect of capitation fees, even though the practice has a higher than average number of elderly patients attracting higher capitation fees. Other factors affecting NHS gross income are:
- the seaside location gives a better than average return so far as concerns temporary resident fees
- the high number of elderly patients causes a lower return on item-of-service fees, such as maternity and contraception, and on target payments
- sessional payments are particularly low and the practice should therefore consider whether improvements can be made in this area.
• The practice recoup the shortfall of NHS gross income by non-NHS activities, which produce 12.6% of their total income.
• Net NHS and non-NHS remuneration at £69 727 per partner and £36.47 per patient is well above intended averages due to non-NHS activities and, in particular, the exceptional control exercised over practice expenses. Expenses per partner are well below national average, even if they have increased over the previous year. The practice seems to have great ability in attracting reimbursement so that their net expenses are particularly low. Cost control has enabled the practice to exceed net NHS remuneration even with a shortfall of gross NHS income.
• The return from practice staff reimbursements (68%) is just below average and shows a fall from the 78.4% achieved in the previous year. The practice clearly saw the need to recruit to cope with work-load, but at a reimbursement level of only £6.34 per patient they may well have an opportunity to renegotiate their staff budget with the HA.
• The return from night visit fees has increased significantly compared with the previous year but is still below average. The increase no doubt corresponds with the decline in locum and deputising costs as the partners perform their own night visits. It is equally clear that the practice has somehow restricted the number of night visits actually performed, which may reflect the geographical location of the practice.

As an overview, the partners may well be satisfied with average earnings per partner of £69 727 before tax. This practice clearly performs well, but as the statistics suggest, there is always room for improvement.

DOCTORS BLACK, WHITE, GREEN, BROWN, ORANGE AND GREY STATISTICS FOR THE YEAR ENDED 30 JUNE 1999

Statistics	National profile 1999	Year ended 1999	Year ended 1998
1 Average patient numbers:			
0–64	8385	7910	7868
65–74	845	920	915
75 and over	715	730	700
	9945	9560	9483
2 Average number of full-time equivalent equity partners	5	5	5
3 Average patients per full-time equivalent partner	1989	1912	1897
4 Gross NHS income per patient	£36.52	£33.56	£31.90
5 Gross practice income per patient (excluding reimbursements)	£42.39	£41.30	£35.36
6 Profit per patient	£27.39	£36.47	£34.19
7 Gross practice income per full-time partner (excluding reimbursements)			
– from NHS	72 638	64 168	60 494
– from other sources	11 674	14 789	6571
	£84 312	£78 957	£67 065
8 Average profit per full-time partner			
– from NHS	49 638	56 667	58 492
– from other sources	4841	13 060	6354
	£54 479	£69 727	£64 846
9 Average expenses per full-time partner			
– from NHS	23 000	7501	2002
– from other sources	6833	1729	217
	£29 833	£9230	£2219
10 Items of service (per patient):			
Night visits	1.61	1.28	1.04
Maternity	1.54	1.32	1.13
Contraception	1.14	0.91	0.62
Vaccinations and immunisations	0.59	0.64	0.61
Temporary residents	0.37	0.64	0.83
Emergency treatment	0.08	0.02	0.03
	£5.33	£4.81	£4.26

DOCTORS BLACK, WHITE, GREEN, BROWN, ORANGE AND GREY
STATISTICS (continued) FOR THE YEAR ENDED 30 JUNE 1999

		1999	1999	1998
11	Sessional pay (per patient):			
	Health promotion	1.48	1.27	1.37
	Minor surgery	0.61	0.29	0.26
	Undergraduate medical students	0.04	0.19	0.29
		£2.13	£1.75	£1.92
12	Child health surveillance fees (per patient)	0.55	0.65	0.63
	Registration fees (per patient)	0.46	0.91	0.90
		£1.01	£1.56	£1.53
13	Practice total income profile (percentage):			
	GMS fees and allowances	56.0	54.7	58.4
	Reimbursements	35.0	32.7	35.3
	Non-GMS income	9.0	12.6	6.3
		100.0%	100.0%	100.0%
14	GMS income profile (percentage):			
	Allowances	16.8	17.7	18.2
	Capitation fees	52.9	50.8	51.7
	Target payments	7.1	9.6	8.5
	Sessional pay	5.8	5.2	6.0
	Items of service	14.9	14.3	13.4
	Other GMS income	2.5	2.4	2.2
		100.0%	100.0%	100.0%
15	Percentage expenses to total income:			
	Staff costs	31.5	21.0	14.2
	Medical expenses	9.5	7.6	9.2
	Premises	6.0	3.0	2.5
	Administration	7.5	1.4	1.4
	Finance	2.5	6.9	9.7
	Depreciation	1.0	0.7	0.4
		58.0%	40.6%	37.4%
16	Percentage staff reimbursement	68.5%	68.0%	78.4%
17	Practice staff reimbursement per patient	£11.57	£6.34	£3.71

Note: (i) Fundholding figures are ignored.
(ii) The national profile in the above example has not been apportioned to take account of the June year-end accounting date.

Figure 12.1   Statistics extracted from a specimen set of accounts

13 Financing a new GP

Most general practices, at some time, face the problem of how to cater for expansion in the practice. Such expansion can arise for a number of reasons: the practice may be in an expanding area with a great deal of new building taking place; it may have attracted patients from other practices by offering better facilities; or the introduction of new and younger partners may have encouraged patients to join who may not otherwise have done so. Some practices, for instance, have found that their popularity is increased by the introduction of a female partner.

If a partner leaves the practice, causing a drop in the number of partners, the remaining doctors must decide whether they need to recruit a new partner. Some practices have reasoned that if, for example, six partners can cater for 12 000 patients at an average of 2000 each, five partners should not have too much trouble in taking on 400 extra patients each. Some practices have indeed chosen to take that course. These tend to be practices made up of younger partners who do not object to taking on an additional workload.

Nevertheless, some partnerships find they cannot continue with their present number of doctors and seek to recruit an additional partner to share the workload. There are a number of ways in which this can be done, and the financial consequences of all options should be considered.

Figure 13.1 compares three options for a four-doctor practice which needs help to cope with its expanding workload. In the year 1998/99, the practice earned a total of £200 000, an average of £50 000 each. For the purpose of these calculations, it is assumed that such items as seniority, PGEA and cost rent allowances are treated as prior charges on profits and they have been excluded from the calculation. The practice has a total of 10 800 patients, or 2700 per partner. The eldest partner, at 45 years of age, still has family commitments; therefore the partnership is reluctant to burden itself with the potential dilution of its profits by taking on an additional partner. It has considered recruiting a locum or an assistant doctor and has estimated the cost of either at £30 000 per annum. It has also considered recruiting an additional partner.

The practice has already been paying out £15 000 per annum to part-time locums, who have worked when required during periods of holidays and sickness. The recruitment of an additional doctor would dispense with this cost.

Locum fees

The partners have been advised that if they appoint a locum, and pay him a regular salary, then they will be required to pay the employer's share of his Class 1 NIC. This would incur an additional (and irrecoverable) cost of about £3000. They would prefer not to do this, and to avoid it must make sure that the locums they employ are assessable to Schedule D tax on their earnings, i.e. they must be effectively self-employed. The cost to the partners of this arrangement would be £30 000, but from this would be deducted the £15 000 presently paid to part-time locums.

A regular locum may not be accepted by the HA as an assistant and would therefore be unable to attract an assistant's allowance.

An assistant

An assistant is an employee of the practice; he or she will be in an employer–employee relationship to the practice, which will be responsible for deducting PAYE tax from the salary and for the employer's share of the Class 1 NIC. At a salary of £30 000 this would represent an additional cost (at 1999/2000 rates) of 12.2% or £3260. The practice would, however, subject to agreement of the HA, be able to attract the assistant's allowance for a non-designated area of £7155 for 1999/2000.

A new partner

The introduction of a new partner is in many ways the most satisfactory solution. The practice will, in theory, save the locum fees previously paid, but will attract another BPA (presently £8256) without any additional costs except the payment to the new partner of his share of the profits. However, the desirability of this option will depend on the new partner's share of the profits and progression to parity. In the example given, it is assumed that he will be recruited at an initial share of 10%, rising to parity over three years by two equal and intermediate steps before achieving parity at 20% of the profits.

An outline of comparative costs is set out in Figure 13.1.

Four full-time GPs; average profits £75 000 after paying locum fees of £15 000; 10 800 patients.

	Present position (1998/99) £	Locum £	New position (1999/2000) Assistant £	Partner £
Partnership profit	300 000	300 000	300 000	300 000
Add: Inflation @ (say) 3%	–	9000	9000	9000
Basic practice allowance	–	–	–	8256
Assistant's allowance	–	–	7155	–
Saving in locum fees (part-time)	–	15 000	15 000	15 000
	300 000	324 000	331 155	332 256
Less: Locum fees	–	30 000	–	–
Assistant's salary	–	–	30 000	–
Class 1 NIC (10%)	–	–	3000	–
	300 000	294 000	298 155	332 256
Profit shares: 4 partners each:				
1998/99	75 000			
1999/2000		73 500	74 539	
New partner @ 10%				33 226 (1)
4 partners (each)				74 758

(1) This share will increase by stages (probably over 3 years) until the new partner achieves parity

Figure 13.1 Comparative costs for a four-doctor practice taking on a locum, assistant or fifth partner

Comparison of results

It may be seen from the calculation in Figure 13.1 that, using the locum option, the partners will each receive a share of the profits of £73 500, which represents a slight fall from their previous year's income. This may be thought worthwhile, bearing in mind the saving in the workload entailed.

The recruitment of an assistant, however, will attract a potential income of £74 539 each, or an increase of about 1%.

The recruitment of a partner will result in a similar rate of increase, but there are other advantages which accrue. The partners would assure the succession of the practice and, if there is a surgery ownership situation, they may be able to pass on a share of this to the incoming partner in due course. Unless there is likely to be a fall in the list sizes, which seems un- likely, the partners will have a continuing average of 2160 patients (somewhat above the national average). The permanence of a new partner is also a guarantee of stability. However, the new partner's share of the profits will rise fairly sharply over a three-year period, and this could reduce the shares of the other partners in real terms unless they are able to attract new sources of income.

14 Joining a practice

The majority of those entering a general practice partnership for the first time will be doing so shortly after completing a general practice vocational training scheme. During training, a practitioner may form an idea of what his ideal practice will be. When the search begins for an ideal practice, it is helpful if the practitioner concerned has decided on a range of features that are considered vital, some features that may be desirable and those elements which, if necessary, may be amended in the light of the opportunities that present themselves.

Choosing a practice

The location of a practice will determine to a significant extent the lifestyles of the GP and the population served. The spectrum ranges from rural dispensing practices, through semi-rural and suburban practices, to inner-city practices serving areas of high social deprivation. The prospective principal must decide which type of practice for which his aptitudes and skills are best suited. The rural practice will almost certainly offer a pleasant environment, perhaps the possibility of participating in the work of a cottage hospital, and the opportunity to become part of the social life of the area. Balanced against this could be the disadvantages of professional isolation, less choice of staff to assist in the running of the practice and reduced opportunity for maintaining close contact with large district general hospitals.

The practitioner seeking an urban practice may be looking for the challenge of serving a population subject to a range of social disadvantages, perhaps the opportunity to become involved in the academic activities of university departments and teaching hospitals, and the greater contact with the profession generally offered by the high GP population in urban areas.

Geographical location may also determine the level of competition for each vacancy. Competition for vacancies in general practice is keen and the competition for particularly attractive vacancies may appear daunting. A practitioner is fortunate if he obtains the first vacancy for which he applies. It is usual for a prospective principal to make a series of applications before being successful. During a period of unsuccessful applications, it is tempting to make compromises over the 'ideal' practice. It is important that the practitioner judges in advance those features over which a compromise is possible and those where he is not prepared to compromise.

How can suitable vacancies be identified? First impressions will be gained from information available from course organisers, HAs or an advertisement. Similarly, a written application will be the first impression that a partnership gains of a candidate. How then should an application for a vacancy in general practice be submitted? As dozens of applications may be submitted, it is important to provide a letter of application and curriculum vitae that tell a practice something about the candidate, and which command its interest.

The curriculum vitae

Studies undertaken by personnel professionals indicate that the average time spent looking at each job application is less than one minute. In that time a judgement is made regarding whether the applicant is suitable for the job being advertised. A curriculum vitae must contain information about personal details and qualifications and experience in medicine.

Personal details should include the following:

- name and address, nationality, date of birth and age
- marital status
- possession of current driving licence
- state of health
- professional qualifications and medical experience, including period of attendance at university and medical school, with details of any distinctions or prizes obtained
- date of full registration with the GMC
- a list of all medical appointments held, starting with the most recent and listing them in reverse chronological order, including any special service such as military or VSO
- details of current employment and availability to enter general practice
- any special experience
- membership or Fellowship of Royal Colleges or Faculties
- other postgraduate qualifications
- details of research or published articles, including special interests pursued while undertaking hospital jobs or general practice vocational training
- interests outside medicine, particularly the gaining of any distinction, in sport for example

- the names, addresses and telephone numbers of referees, who must always include the candidate's trainer and course organiser.

A curriculum vitae should be professionally typed and clearly set out, with appropriate margins or spacings left for those who shortlist and interview to make comments and notes. The letter accompanying the curriculum vitae should be handwritten, legible and provide a personal perspective on the reasons for the application, including the candidate's particular interest in the practice vacancy and the location of the practice.

An application may result in one or more interviews at the practice. A good practice will provide a practice profile in advance to give you basic information that can be added to when attending the practice for interview. It is not unusual for an applicant to be subjected to an initial interview which provides the practice with the opportunity to draw up a short list for final selection.

Questions to ask

What questions should a doctor ask when invited to an interview? Of paramount importance is information regarding the partners with whom, if successful, the doctor may be working for the rest of his professional life. The candidate should find out how many there are, their ages, how the partnership vacancy arose, how the partnership conducts its management of the practice and what sort of new partner they are seeking.

An immediate impression of the premises will be gained on the first visit. If it is a health centre, the doctor should ascertain the lease arrangements with the HA. If the property is owned by the partnership, questions will be needed about the incoming partner's obligations with regard to the financing of the premises and the purchase of the capital share of those premises (see Chapters 15 and 16). The doctor should satisfy himself that the premises, furnishings and equipment within the practice appear in good condition, that there are facilities for the staff and that the practice as a whole is equipped to deal with its list of patients. He should also enquire about any particular difficulties with the premises, such as a lack of parking space for the partners.

It is important to learn about the practice staff: how many staff are employed by the practice and do the staff include a practice nurse or other health professionals? Is there a practice administrator or manager, and does the practice issue formal written contracts and job descriptions for its staff? Are there staff who are attached to the practice, for example a health visitor or a social worker? What is the usual method of communicating with staff members? Does any one partner have a particular responsibility for staff and personnel matters? The candidate will note how the staff treated him when he first arrived at the practice.

Questions regarding financial matters are dealt with in detail elsewhere. A doctor will wish to be satisfied that the financial affairs of the practice are in good order and accordingly will require some idea about the accounts within the practice, the main sources of income of the practice and any major financial obligations which the practice is taking on or may take on in the near future.

An applicant for a vacancy should find out about the partnership arrangements: it is important to establish whether there is a written partnership agreement and what it states. A practice without a valid agreement may be one to avoid.

No practice operates in total isolation and it is therefore important to establish the relationships the practice has with the HA, the LMC, local hospitals and their consultants, other practices and the social services department of the local authority. If the area is unfamiliar, it is important to find out about the local housing market, ease of travel, schooling, banks and shopping facilities.

The interview

Generally, the most difficult hurdle in the process of joining a new practice is the interview. An invitation to interview indicates that an applicant has passed the first hurdle and that the written application has succeeded in 'selling' that doctor. At the interview, the process of selling oneself continues, but it is equally important that the interview creates a two-way process by which the partners can judge the applicant and the applicant can reflect on whether he wishes to join that partnership. A good interview will be a relaxed and friendly affair, but sufficiently businesslike to ensure that candidates can be properly assessed and interviewers judged. First impressions count. The candidate who is dressed for the occasion and is positive and direct in manner will impress at the outset. Preparation is also vital and, where the applicant has been sent material in advance, it should be obvious whether the material has been read and understood. It is particularly important that the candidate should be ready to answer questions where the application reveals an earlier interest or commitment to a career in hospital medicine, or where there appear to be unexplained gaps in the employment chronology. Candidates will always be asked if they have any questions themselves and it is common sense to prepare two or three questions in advance. This should not inhibit asking questions during the course of the interview, provided that this does not mean that the interviewing panel are unable to get through all the questions they have planned to ask.

Throughout the interview, the main question that the interviewers and the applicant will have at the back of their minds is 'Can I get on with this person?'. The answer to that question will arise from the manner and conduct at the interview, from the way in which the applicants 'come over', how open they are, how truthful they are and how committed they appear to the vacancy on offer. Where part of the interviewing process involves the applicant's spouse, it is important to ensure that the applicant and spouse do not put across conflicting messages to the partnership. There is no point in a doctor applying for a post emphasising the advantage placed on the value of life in a rural practice if the spouse has interests and commitments which can be fulfilled only in an urban environment.

If successful, the new partner will be subject to a probationary period, commonly called a period of mutual assessment. This may last for between three and 12 months, and provides for a period in which neither side to a new agreement is making a final commitment. The new partner has a chance to measure his expectations of the practice against the reality, and the partnership taking in a new doctor will be able to judge whether the interviewing process has successfully identified the correct candidate for the post. Although it is rare for the period of mutual assessment not to lead to continuing partnership with the incoming doctor, it provides an important safeguard for all concerned and can avoid the trauma and difficulty associated with the departure of a partner.

15 Calculating the partners' drawings

In all partnerships there must be a system of withdrawing funds from the practice account by the partners, so that income can be passed to their own accounts for personal use. Doctors, like all other sections of the community, have their personal living expenses to finance and there must be a regular and controlled means of transferring funds to them.

For employees, such as hospital doctors, GP registrars and consultants, this is not a problem. Their salaries will normally be paid to them at the end of each month, having undergone all necessary deductions. GPs, however, are not employees; as we have seen, they are self-employed individuals and, as partners, they have a responsibility to each other. One of these is to ensure that funds passed to them from time to time are in keeping both with their profit-sharing ratios and all other known factors.

Unfortunately, incorrect terminology is often used; it is highly misleading when doctors refer to the monthly amounts paid to them as their 'salary'. This is not the case and the fact cannot be emphasised too strongly. The word 'salary' has all manner of unfortunate connotations in this context, not least being the manner in which the income is taxed, and it is better to avoid the term if at all possible.

It is no exaggeration to say that the periodic calculation of partnership drawings is one of the financial procedures which regularly causes most difficulties to GPs in partnership. Many doctors feel that knowledge of their incomes is of such a confidential nature that it cannot be delegated to a member of their staff. These calculations are therefore, in many cases, done by one of the partners themselves. Fortunately, attitudes are changing and, in an increasing number of cases, such drawings calculations are done by a responsible practice manager.

Rather different problems concern the single-handed practitioner. He has no partners to worry about and the money he earns is his own, subject of course to making prudent provisions for income tax and other matters. He may, however, be well advised to pass all his professional transactions through a separate practice bank account and to transfer monthly such sums as can reasonably be set aside into his private bank account for his own use.

Drawings calculations should be made correctly and accurately, if partners are to avoid feeling they are receiving more or less than their proper entitlement, and in order to avoid disparities in their current accounts at the end of each financial year.

Whether drawings have been properly calculated or not will become evident when the annual partnership accounts are prepared; any differences between the current accounts of the partners will then become apparent. Steps should be taken to see that such errors do not recur and that the balances are adjusted by subsequent and 'one-off' adjustments to drawings. An example of these current account balances is shown in Chapter 10 on practice accounts.

There are probably as many different systems of drawings by partners as there are fingers on one's hands. Whatever system is used, it is essential that it is operated properly. The simplest system would apply in a two-man partnership sharing profits equally, so that both doctors could withdraw identical amounts. In practice, that is likely to be the exception rather than the rule. In virtually all cases, complex adjustments will be made for differing rates of seniority awards, superannuation payments, added years contributions, loan interest charges, national insurance, repayments of leave advance and similar adjustments.

The system which is perhaps most widely used in partnerships is the 'month-end' or 'quarter-end' system, under which partners are paid at the end of each month, and adjustments made quarterly to take into consideration the factors mentioned above. While it is acceptable that payments at the end of the two intermediate months may be made in partnership ratios, the full measure of adjustments must be made at the end of the quarter. This is illustrated by the example shown in Figure 15.1. This shows a four-doctor partnership, Drs A, B, C and D, the three senior partners having a share of 28% and a new partner, Dr D, with a share of 16%. Drs A and B are both paying for added years (A); all the partners are paying leave advances (B); while Dr D has a loan from the GP Finance Corporation (C). Drs A, B, C and D have seniority awards at varying rates (D). The figures shown are for illustration purposes only and it should not be assumed that these will apply to partnerships in practice.

In computing the total amount to be distributed, it is normal to find the balance available on the partnership bank account (E), either by reference to the bank statements at the end of the quarter or, more preferably and where adequate and accurate records are kept, by referring to the balance in hand as shown in the practice cash book. There should be retained from the amount the estimated expenditure to run the practice during the succeeding months (F), and the balance will then be available for distribution (G).

It should be remembered that, at the same time as this distribution is made, certain deductions have been made from the quarterly HA remuneration and, similarly, certain additions will have been included (*see* Box 15.1). It

Drs A, B, C and D	Total £	Dr A 28%	Dr B 28%	Dr C 28%	Dr D 16%
Balance in partnership					
bank account (E)	13 000				
Less:					
retain on hand (F)	4500				
For distribution (G)	8500				
Add deductions:					
Superannuation	540				
Added years (A)	120				
Leave advance (B)	1200				
GPFC loan (C)	125				
Monthly on account	10 000	11 985			
		20 485			
Less additional income:					
Seniority (D)	2800				
For allocation (in partnership ratios)	17 685	4952	4952	4952	2829
Add:					
Seniority (D)	2800	1000	1000	400	400
	20 485	5952	5952	5352	3229
Less.					
Superannuation	540	150	150	150	90
Added years (A)	120	75	45		300
Leave advance (B)	1200	300	300	300	125
GPFC loan (C)	125	1985	525	495	450	515
	18 500	5427	5457	4902	2714
Less: paid monthly on account	10 000	2800	2800	2800	1600
Net withdrawals	8500	2627	2657	2102	1114

Figure 15.1 Calculation of quarterly drawings, October 1999

Box 15.1: Details of likely items to be adjusted on periodic drawings calculations

Income

- seniority awards
- PGEA
- notional rent allowance (where to be distributed in different ratios to partnership shares)

Outgoings

- superannuation contributions: standard
- added years and unreduced lump sum
- NIC
- repayment of leave advances
- GPFC (or other loan repayments and interest)
- transfers to income tax reserve

---

is necessary to reverse these entries before arriving at the total allocation for the quarter and then to allocate the proper amounts to each of the four partners.

It may also be that certain of the partners do not own the surgery premises and they will not be entitled to share in any notional rent allowances in respect of the building. A detailed examination of the quarterly HA statement should be made to ensure that all items of this nature are taken into account.

Equalised drawings systems

Many partnerships prefer to operate a system of equalised drawings, under which a full year's net income is estimated and divided into equal amounts for distribution to the partners. Provided that all proper adjustments have been made, this regular monthly withdrawal can be paid to the partners' personal bank accounts by standing order.

This system allows a partner to estimate his regular monthly income, for the purpose of his personal family budget, and also avoids the constant calculation and issue of monthly cheques. The system is illustrated in Figure 15.2, for a four-doctor partnership with varying rates of superannuation, seniority, added years and other items. This calculation is normally

	Total	Dr A (28%) £	Dr B (28%) £	Dr C (24%) £	Dr D (20%) £
Estimated partnership profits for year	90 000	25 200	25 200	21 600	18 000
Seniority awards	7400	3900	2000	–	1500
Total income (est.) (1)	97 400	29 100	27 200	21 600	19 500
Deductions					
Superannuation (est.)	5600	1600	1500	1300	1200
Added years	1300	800	300	200	–
Outside appts (est.)	100	–	20	80	–
National insurance (est.)					
Class I (appointments)	100	–	–	100	–
Class II (stamps)	960	240	240	240	240
Repayment of leave advance	4824	1206	1206	1206	1206
Repayment of loans (GPFC)	1300	–	–	500	800
	14 184	3846	3266	3626	3446
Income tax reserve transfers	18 000	6500	5500	4000	2000
Total outgoings (2)	32 184	10 346	8766	7626	5446
Net (1–2)	65 216	18 754	18 434	13 974	14 054
Monthly	5434	1563	1536	1164	1171
(rounded down)	5415	1560	1530	1160	1165

Figure 15.2 Calculation of equalised drawings for the year to June 1999

made on a tax year basis, so that a reserve can be made for the self-assessment tax liabilities of the individual partners.

The detailed preparation of such an equalised drawings system will normally be done by the partnership accountant, who should have the required detailed information available to him, and who will be in a position to calculate the tax reserve to be operated during any given period.

The use of income tax reserve accounts

We have looked at the manner in which drawings calculations are made and, ideally, these will take into account the tax liabilities of the individual partners.

The rationale for maintaining separate funds to pay future tax liabilities has been largely thrown into question by the virtue of the fact that, under the new self-assessment regulations, from 1997/98 there have been no further tax liabilities on partnerships, with the liability falling due in the names of the individual partners. Now that there is no possibility of partners being held liable for the unpaid tax liabilities of their colleagues, some practices feel that the retention of such monies in tax reserve accounts is no longer necessary. However, many practices have opted to continue to put money aside in the prescribed manner, largely due to the comfort of knowing that funds are available when these liabilities fall due.

Under the self-assessment system also, tax is now payable on 31 January and 31 July annually (see Chapter 23). Where the practice decides to maintain separate funds of this nature, these should be done under control, with the necessary professional advice, to ensure that funds are available when the tax falls due for settlement. The timescale for the operation of such a reserve is important and to a great degree depends on the estimates of future liabilities being received as early as possible within each separate tax year.

The reserve should be held physically separate from the main partnership funds, either in a building society or bank deposit account, and the periodic interest divided between the partners in proportion to their shares of the balance on hand. It should preferably be transferred by means of a monthly standing order from the main partnership bank account, on a tax year basis so that for, say, the 1999/2000 year, 12 monthly transfers would be made, from the end of April 1999 until March 2000.

A typical reserve is illustrated in Figure 15.3, which shows a four-doctor practice with an estimated liability for 1999/2000 of £18 000. This could have been calculated in January or February 1999 and may require some amendment to take account of amended allowances and tax rates which have been introduced in the 1998 Budget. Interest will be credited to the various partners in proportions to their different contributions.

	Annual tax liability 1999/2000 £	Monthly reserve April 1999–March 2000 £
Dr W	6000	495
Dr X	5000	410
Dr Y	4750	390
Dr Z	2250	185
	18 000	1480

The monthly transfer can be slightly less than 1/12 of the annual liability, due to interest which will be credited to the account.

Figure 15.3   Income tax reserve

16   Surgery finance

One of the factors that sets the NHS GP apart from other sections of the business community, including NHS dentists, is the manner in which the business premises are organised and financed. Detailed rules are contained in paragraph 51 of the SFA.

The provision of surgery premises is likely to fall under one of five categories:

1 rented from a private landlord
2 rented from the local authority
3 a health centre occupancy
4 owned by the partners
5 a cost rent development.

Some multi-surgery practices may have premises under two or more of these categories.

As discussed in Chapter 3, a relatively high level of GPs' expenses are refunded directly to the practice, and other expenses are refunded indirectly through the annual remuneration award. For surgery premises, however, a separate set of rules exists. It is necessary for GPs to understand these fully, as regards both rented and owner-occupied surgeries.

Rented surgeries

A GP who rents a surgery from a landlord has the right to recover the rent from the HA. Normally, this will be repaid fully, except in cases where the whole of the premises is not given over to NHS work. If, for instance, part of the property is sublet to a private tenant, a refund would not be made for that proportion of the rent. If the building is in combined use, partly for domestic or other use and the remaining part for the practice, an apportionment of the refund is normally calculated by the District Valuer.

Health centre accommodation

GPs practising from health centres should be aware that their rent (together with rates, water rates, etc.) will not, in effect, be paid from their own sources and refunded, but will be internally recorded by the health authority.

In the case of both health centres and rented surgeries, care must be taken to see that the rent paid (or notional rent) is accurately shown on one side of the accounts and the (notional) refund on the other. This is to ensure that, if these accounts are selected by the Review Body for the 'sampling process', the GPs' expenses will be maximised so that they do not artificially depress the level of average expenses indirectly refunded in the annual pay award. This is particularly important for health centre practices, and the accountant drawing up the accounts should understand the necessity for this exercise.

In many cases, however, surgeries are not rented from a third party, but are owned by the doctor(s), either in sole practice or in partnership. In this case, a rent allowance is paid to the doctors in order to recompense them for the use of their privately owned surgery for NHS purposes.

The notional rent allowance

Notional rent is paid on surgeries that are owner-occupied, but either are not new or have been erected or developed in a manner that falls outside the scope of the cost rent scheme (*see* below). Notional rent payments for owner-occupiers, in respect of separate premises and/or premises forming part of a residence, are determined after assessment by the District Valuer according to a valuation based on the current market rent which may reasonably be expected to be paid for the premises.

The agreed amount is then paid in full to the GP(s), usually at quarterly or monthly intervals. Every effort should be made to improve cash flow (*see* Chapter 6) to ensure that the rent allowance is received monthly.

Notional rent is valued at triennial intervals, normally resulting in an increase in the rent allowance, and most practices show a steady increase in the rent allowance over the years. If they are not satisfied, the doctors have a right of appeal to the Secretary of State. This is frequently exercised and it is believed that, in the majority of cases, such appeals are successful. In some cases, however, due to the property recession, valuations have fallen. This is dealt with more fully in Chapter 29.

The council tax, being a tax on property, can be included in claims for refunds of direct expenses or personal expenses.

There are several other property-related reimbursements, which are dealt with in Chapter 3.

Partnerships

The property-owing partnership is now extremely common, although many of the major new surgery developments are only suitable or viable for larger group practices, or a combination of practices.

It is important to consider the effect of ownership on the organisation of the practice finances.

It is common for such surgeries to be owned by the partners in other than their standard profit-sharing ratios. In a partnership of six doctors, two might be part-time or partially retired GPs who do not wish to partake in the surgery ownership, which would leave ownership in four shares.

The receipt of the cost or notional rent allowance, which is effectively the return on the partners' investment, should be credited to the surgery owners and not to the other partners. Similarly, the cost of servicing a loan should be dealt with on the same basis. This is illustrated in the accounts shown in Chapter 10, by the inclusion of separate notes (2 and 15) showing the allocation of such items as a prior share of profit.

See also Chapter 17: Capital Accounts.

Improvement grants

Grants are available for the improvement of surgery premises – currently up to a third of the total cost – although these are subject to 'cash limiting' by HAs in the same way as cost rent and other refunds.

Such grants are normally paid on completion of an improvement project, but improvements should only be embarked upon with the prior agreement of the HA.

One condition of claiming the improvement grant is that the same expenditure must not be claimed for income tax purposes. Whilst many improvements or alterations to the structure of the building will be of a capital nature and will not in any event attract capital allowances, there are certain circumstances in which tax relief could be claimed on identical expenditure, and a decision will have to be made as to which of these is preferable.

Whilst each case must be considered strictly on its individual merits, the present level of tax and capital allowances rates means that, for most such projects, it is more beneficial to claim the improvement grant and relinquish any potential tax relief.

Taxation

The rent allowance is paid to GPs on the use of privately owned surgeries to see NHS patients; it is unconnected with 'rent' in the generally accepted sense of the term, and it is essential that for taxation purposes this principle is understood. It is incorrect to treat the allowance as the private, unearned income of the doctor(s) and to enter it in the property section of their self-assessment tax returns; otherwise this can have a radical effect on the way the income is taxed.

The income should be treated as part of the practice profits, and allocated between the partners in ratios applicable to their shares of ownership for the property, not in those in which residual partnership profits are divided.

Relief for interest paid

Interest on surgery loans is allowed in full for tax purposes, and extreme care must be taken to see that only partners owning shares in the surgery premises obtain relief on the interest paid. Such relief is granted on the same basis that applies to all other expenses a GP incurs (*see* Chapter 24).

It is common, in cases of new surgery projects, for interest to be 'rolled up', i.e. not paid during the period of the surgery development but added to the loan for payment at a future date. This interest is also fully allowable on the same basis, but must be shown as an item of expenditure in the practice accounts. It may, however, be possible to re-organise the loan so that further tax benefit to the GP is made available (*see* Chapter 18).

The cost rent scheme

In many cases during recent years, surgeries have been developed under a scheme introduced in the mid-1970s, which has provided new and vastly improved surgery accommodation for NHS patients.

The cost rent scheme offers a unique opportunity to acquire a valuable capital asset without significant capital outlay. No other profession, either inside or outside the NHS, is offered a scheme of a similar nature, the advantages of which are shown in Box 16.1.

Yet, surprisingly, many doctors have still not felt able to take advantage of it, in many cases being inhibited by the relatively large costs involved. This is unfortunate because the introduction of cash limiting from 1 April 1990 has in some cases succeeded in deferring or aborting new projects.

> **Box 16.1: Benefits of the cost rent scheme**
>
> 1 Tax-free capital appreciation.
> 2 Increasing income.
> 3 Taxation benefits.

A concise account of the scheme, and the manner in which it operates, is given in *Making Sense of the Cost Rent Scheme*, published by Radcliffe Medical Press. This chapter looks at some of the implications of a non-financial nature for doctors embarking on a project for surgery development.

As we have seen, GPs who do not own their premises are eligible for reimbursement of the rent and rates paid on the premises, provided the HA is satisfied that the use of existing premises, the enlargement of premises, or a move to new premises, is justified in the interests of the NHS.

On the other hand, GPs who own their own premises are normally paid a rent allowance (as opposed to a refund) based upon the estimated rental value of the property. As an alternative to receiving a 'notional rent' reimbursement, however, some practices choose to apply for reimbursement related to the cost of providing purpose-built premises, or their equivalent. This is known as 'cost rent', provided that the project falls within one of the following categories:

1 the building of completely new premises
2 the acquisition of premises for substantial modification
3 the substantial modification of existing practice premises.

The scheme does *not* provide for the direct reimbursement of interest paid, or payable, on borrowing facilities arranged to meet the costs of a project; and it cannot be stressed too strongly that, before entering into a financial commitment or other obligation, GPs should ensure that the project is financially viable. They must be able to meet the costs of servicing and repaying the loan from the receipt of the cost rent allowance, other practice income and/or private means.

As the name implies, the cost rent scheme calculates the rent allowance by reference to the total cost of a development project, to which a percentage factor is applied. If, for instance, the total agreed cost of a project is £900 000, and there is a 7% fixed rate of cost rent in force at the time, the annual reimbursement will be £63 000.

There are four main components in the cost of such a project:

1 the cost of buying the land
2 the cost of erection (building contract)
3 professional and architects' fees
4 bridging interest.

GPs should, at the outset of a project and before taking on any financial commitment, seek the HA's agreement to the proposals 'in principle', and ascertain the priority accorded to the project in the authority's forward programme for premises improvement, including any provisional estimate of when cost reimbursement can be expected for the scheme (SFA, paragraph 51.51). In other words, not only must approval be obtained for the project, but an indication must be given as to whether the HA is in a position to designate sufficient funds for the scheme.

The cost rent limits

The maximum amount that may be spent on a new surgery project is strictly limited with respect to building costs.

Many developing practices have found it virtually impossible to build surgeries within these limits and have been left to finance a significant shortfall out of current earnings. This situation has to some degree been resolved by the introduction of variations in limits by means of the banding and other systems.

Location factors

A system of banding based on building cost location factors applicable to each HA area in the UK is in force.

Total cost calculation

Once all the figures are available, it should be possible to establish with some degree of accuracy the likely level of cost rent reimbursement. Figure 16.1 shows a typical (if simplified) calculation for a practice in Berkshire to which a factor of 1.04 applies. It illustrates a typical situation where the proceeds from the cost rent allowance (£55 250) are identical to the interest on the loan finance, but not the annual cost of capital repayment.

This problem could be deferred by a capital repayment 'holiday' for the first few years of the loan, in the expectation that when capital repayments become due these will be covered by an increase in income due to a conversion to a 'notional rent' basis.

Fixed and variable allowances

Once the final cost rent limit has been calculated by the HA, the amount of the cost rent reimbursement is calculated by applying to that limit the prescribed percentage as notified by the DoH to the authority. There are two percentage rates, one variable and the other fixed. The variable rate of reimbursement is reviewed annually in April (6.5% up to 31 March 2000), whereas the fixed rate of reimbursement (6.5% per annum at the time of going to press) is set quarterly.

The variable rate of reimbursement is applied to every project *except* in the following circumstances when the fixed rate applies:

1 where GPs are financing the building scheme wholly or mainly with their own money
2 where they are financing it wholly or mainly with a loan acquired on fixed rate terms.

In both cases, either the input of the GPs' own monies or the draw-down of a fixed rate loan, must be for the majority of the total cost of the project.

		£	£
1	Site (cost or District Valuer's valuation, whichever is the lower)		120 000
2	Building cost (subject to cost rent limits)	475 000	
	Adjust: for location factor (1.04)	19 000	
			494 000
			614 000
3	VAT @ 17.5% on £599 750 (see Chapter 30)		107 450
4	Architects' fees, etc.*	70 610	
	VAT (17.5%)	12 357	
			82 967
5	Bridging interest		45 583
			850 000
	Cost rent reimbursement at variable rate (6.5%)		55 250

* Architects' fees at 11.5% of building cost + VAT

Figure 16.1 Calculation of the cost rent allowance on a typical surgery development project

The SFA allows for situations where GPs finance the scheme wholly or mainly with a fixed rate loan, *but* with the option to switch to a variable rate at a future date. In such cases, the fixed rate of reimbursement will apply until the GP exercises the option and then the prevailing prescribed variable rate will be applied by the committee.

This ruling brings greater flexibility to the scheme and may be used to protect the GPs, or at least give them an advantage in times of rising interest rates. They can benefit from short-term fixed rate schemes made available by financial institutions, yet retain the ability to switch at a future date when there is a higher variable rate of reimbursement. The rate of reimbursement should be calculated by applying the approved prescribed percentage to the approved costs of the scheme; in the case of the variable rate, this is adjusted annually, but the fixed rate will not change regardless of general market conditions or rates.

Unless the aforementioned option is available, GPs should think carefully before committing themselves to borrowing at fixed rates. Long-term fixed rate borrowing may involve taking out an endowment policy and it should be asked whether the lending rate will be fixed for the duration of the loan. Thought should also be given to the situation of an incoming partner, who may be financially worse off by having a fixed rate of reimbursement, whilst having to borrow at a much higher variable rate to buy into a practice.

Advice should, at an early stage, be sought from the HA and the practice's financial advisers.

When to change to notional rent

Paragraph 51.52.21 of the SFA acknowledges that it is unlikely, initially, that the current market rate will produce a more favourable reimbursement than cost rent.

Cost rent will continue to be paid until the premises (or a significant part of them) cease to be used for practice purposes, or the GP chooses on a review to change to current market rent. A review can be requested:

1 every three years from the operative date to the cost rent when the premises are owned by the GPs, or
2 for premises leased by the GP, when a review of rent payable is due under the terms of the lease, or a new lease is entered into at the end of the full term of the existing lease.

Notional rent will be reviewed at triennial intervals after the switch from cost rent. No mention is made in the SFA of a reversal back to cost rent.

The decision to switch from cost rent to notional rent depends on several factors. Clearly, notional rent must exceed rent, and in the longer term the GP may feel relatively safe in the knowledge that property values and rents have, with few exceptions, risen each year. Nonetheless, at the time of the review consideration should be given, before authorising the change-over, to the amount of the increased reimbursement compared with forecasts for interest rates, the economic and political climates, and the period to the next review of the prescribed variable rate. The benefit of a higher rate of notional rent reimbursement now would fade if, during the ensuing three years, the variable rate rose to dizzy heights as each annual review reflected rising rates in general.

The final judgement

Any cost rent project must be judged essentially as a long-term investment. It is unlikely that any GP will realise a substantial benefit in the short term.

When all the information is available, a financial appraisal should be produced, which will give the GPs some idea of the likely surplus or shortfall. Figure 16.2 sets out a simplified version of such a statement.

	£	£
Total cost		850 000
Cost rent allowance (6.5% variable)		55 250
Loan repayments:		
Annual interest (6.5%)	55 250 (1)	
Capital repayments (25 years)	34 000	
		89 250
Total annual shortfall		34 000
Per partner (in a 6 partner practice)		5667

(1) Assumed to be identical to rate of reimbursement.

Figure 16.2 What will it cost (excluding taxation)?

17 Capital accounts

There are few topics concerning the finances of the medical partnership which cause such consternation and misunderstanding as the concept of capital accounts and the contributions incoming partners are required to make. Despite the regular stream of articles in the medical press, explaining various aspects of capital accounts, there remains a significant lack of understanding on the part of the young partner who may regard himself as still an employee, either of the HA or the practice, and fail to realise the concept of investment in a business and of the returns to be made from it.

Capital is the oil on which any business runs; without it, a business, for lack of sufficient facility to run its business operations, will inevitably wither and die. To that extent, a medical practice, of whatever type, is effectively no different, except in scale, from the major company or the corner shop.

Capital is effectively the investment by the partners in their business (i.e. the medical practice) and without an adequate supply of capital the business will not survive. We see below exactly how this capital can be made up and how it can be contributed.

This concept of investment in the capital of a business is not unique to medical practices. A multinational company needs to raise capital to develop its potential and finance its current operations, and this is normally done through share issues or loans from banks or finance houses. GPs running a practice, often with a turnover in excess of £1 million a year, must also finance their business operations, surgery development and numerous items of capital equipment, furniture, etc., required to run the practice.

There are two sources of finance available to the GP: loans from outside sources (a bank, GPFC, etc.) or personal resources – either private funds, which may have been borrowed, or restrictions of future drawings. It is more efficient in financial terms if capital comes from the personal resources of the partners rather than from constant and expensive borrowing from the bank, unless it is absolutely necessary.

The various components of capital are shown in Box 17.1 and are discussed in this chapter.

Box 17.1: The capital of a medical partnership: components

1 property capital: net equity in surgery buildings

2 other (fixed asset) capital: investment in furniture, fixtures, fittings, equipment, computers, office machinery, etc.

3 working capital: the net current assets of the practice

2 and 3 can be simplified to fixed capital

Property (or surgery) capital

This applies to surgery-owning practices only. In the case of the financing of surgery developments or the acquisition of shares of equity by a new partner, the money involved will normally be financed by outside sources of borrowing. The initial investment by the GPs will be quite small. Indeed, in many surgery projects, there is 100% financing from the bank. However, the partners' contribution will tend to increase with time due to appreciation in property values and through capital repayments of the loan.

The situation arising on the retirement of an outgoing partner and the introduction of a new partner, where it is proposed to make a sale from the retiring to the incoming partner, is shown in Figure 17.1. The practice developed a new surgery in 1990 at a cost of £250 000, which was wholly borrowed so that there was no initial contribution by the partners. The first change in ownership took place in 1999; the valuation had increased to £400 000, with the loan having been partially repaid and standing at

	1990 £	1999 £
Original cost, 1990	250 000	
Valuation: 31 March 1999		400 000
Less: balance of outstanding loan	250 000	210 000
Equity	–	190 000
One-fifth share	–	38 000
Equity has built up due to:		
Surplus on revaluation (£400K – £250K)		150 000
Part repayment of loan (£250K – £210K)		40 000
		190 000

Figure 17.1 Surgery capital: calculation of partnership share

£210 000. This established the equity in the surgery building at £190 000, which is the basis on which all calculations should be made. The outgoing partner has a one-fifth share from which he would reasonably expect to receive a sum of £38 000. An incoming partner should expect to contribute on the same basis. It can be seen from this example how equity has built up over this seven-year period.

One aspect of surgery capital, which is represented by the equity in the surgery building, is that it is frequently owned by the partners in different proportions to those in which they share practice profits. In a typical partnership, there may be six partners, one of whom is a partially retired GP who has sold his share of the surgery, and another a part-time doctor who is unable to buy a share; the four remaining partners own the surgery, possibly equally, although this may not be the same means by which they share profits from the practice.

In medical partnerships, this causes no undue problems of principle; the proceeds from the surgery ownership, which in practice will be the notional or cost rent allowance together with any other small rentals the practice might receive, less the interest and the surgery loan, should be credited to the surgery-owning partners. It is normal to deal with this by inclusion of a separate allocation in the annual accounts. Only by this means can the surgery-owning partners receive the correct return on their investment in the surgery premises, as opposed to their colleagues who have made no such contribution.

The term 'negative equity' has come into use to denote the situation applying where the loan on a surgery building is higher than the current valuation. Where this applies it is strongly recommended that specialist professional advice is sought.

Other (fixed asset) capital

Apart from the surgery, there will almost certainly be additional capital assets employed by the practice, which it is necessary to record as capital in the books of the partnership and which the partners can expect to exchange among themselves for value on changes in either the constitution of the partnership or in profit-sharing ratios.

These assets will normally consist of items owned by the practice as a whole: furniture (desk, chairs, tables, filing cabinets, etc.); fixtures and fittings (heating installations, plumbing fittings, fixed shelving and filing areas, etc.); medical and surgical equipment (X-ray machines, etc.); office machinery and equipment (telephone installations, computers, copying machines, etc.). In a sizeable practice this could add up to several thousand pounds, and it is normal for a retiring partner to take his share of this on retirement and for the incoming partner to purchase a share of it.

Unlike the surgery building, the return from these assets cannot be quantified exactly; they are, in effect, assets from which the practice earns its income and profits, so that it is reasonable for such assets to be divided in the same ratios as those in which the partners share practice profits.

It is standard and recommended practice for a valuation to be taken when changes in partnership occur. If, for instance, a value of £5000 was placed on fixed assets, the retiring partner could reasonably expect to receive a one-fifth share, i.e. £1000. However, an incoming partner may not be asked to contribute to the same degree if entering at a lower ratio, say 12%, and moving to parity over several years. At 12%, his contribution would only be £600. The remainder should be contributed, normally by drawings adjustments, over the period to parity.

Working capital

The concept of working capital, normally represented by the net current assets of the partnership, is probably the most difficult for incoming partners to understand. Working capital involves less obvious assets, such as those held in cash and debts due to the practice. New partners frequently express surprise when they are asked to contribute to these current assets, although they are part of the legitimate capital of the business from which they earn their income.

In Figure 17.2, the working capital requirement at a given date of a dispensing practice is shown as net current assets of £50 000. At any given date, the practice may be required to hold a fairly large stock of drugs; there may at times be substantial funds due to the practice from the HA and other sources, which it must finance from its own means; and there will be amounts owed by the practice to outside creditors, probably for

Current assets:	£
Stock of dispensing drugs	40 000
Sundry debtors	25 000
Cash at bank	2 500
Cash in hand	50
	67 550
Less: Sundry creditors	17 550
Net current assets	50 000

Figure 17.2   Working capital: net current assets

drug supplies, etc. An incoming partner commencing on a starting share of 12% of the profits could reasonably expect to pay in the same proportion of that amount, i.e. £6000. In the case of a large dispensing practice, it is normal for this to be done by an initial introduction of funds, at the same time as the fixed assets are purchased. In the case of a smaller practice with a reduced capital requirement, the partners may be prepared to accept a gradual build-up of funds due to the restrictions of drawings over an agreed period.

Retiring partners

For partners retiring from practice, who wish to recover the capital invested by them in the practice, the process is relatively easy with respect to the surgery and other capital. Valuations are placed on the assets and the gross value or equity calculated. The calculation of the working capital normally has to wait until the next partnership accounts are prepared so that the amount can be accurately assessed. The partnership deed should lay down in strict terms the manner in which this capital is to be paid over to a retiring partner or the executors of a deceased partner.

Where fixed capital amounts are in operation, the process is a great deal easier, as retiring partners are then fully aware of the extent of their capital investment.

Goodwill

The sale and purchase of goodwill in NHS general practices is illegal and is prohibited under the National Health Service Act. Unlike their colleagues in the dental services, NHS GPs are not deemed to hold any value of goodwill and it cannot be passed, either in specific terms or as 'hidden goodwill', upon changes in partnership. GPs held to have participated in such transactions can be treated severely by the medical authorities.

This prohibition on the sale and purchase of goodwill does not apply to private practices, which are able to transact such business without hindrance.

Fixed capital accounts

Some partnerships express a preference for having their capital calculated on a fixed sum, intended to represent their investment in both the fixed assets and working capital of the practice. This system has a number of advantages:

- by more exactly quantifying the required capital investment by each partner, it facilitates the introduction of new partners
- for similar reasons, it is easier to calculate the capital due to an outgoing partner
- it ensures that the balances on the partners' current accounts at the end of the year represent undrawn profits which can be paid over to them
- it facilitates the organisation of loan finance to provide the most tax-efficient result for each partner. This is discussed more fully in Chapter 18.

It is normal for these fixed capital amounts to be allocated between partners in profit-sharing ratios. Thus, whilst the overall level of capital might not change, the allocation between individual partners may be changed in accordance with revised profit-sharing ratios, e.g. when a junior partner progresses to parity.

From the amounts set out in Chapter 10, the balance sheet indicates that the overall fixed capital has been set at £80 000. The allocations between individual partners (Note 21) are equivalent to their shares of the profit.

18 Efficient capital planning

On numerous occasions, GPs, as partners in their businesses, are required to fund fairly large capital contributions, and this chapter examines how partners can:

- organise the capital of their practice in such a way that it will remain constant from year to year (and how this figure can be calculated)
- reorganise a substantial surgery mortgage to maximise tax benefits
- reorganise their private loan arrangements to 'unlock' some or all of the capital, again for tax benefit.

Fixed capital accounts

We have seen in Chapter 17 (p. 123) how some partnerships can reorganise their capital in such a manner that a fixed sum is quantified, which represents an investment by the partners in the fixed assets and working capital of the practice. Page 128 sets out the advantages in doing so.

In the specimen practice accounts on pages 66–81 the balance sheet (p. 70) shows the overall fixed capital of the practice at £80 000. This is calculated by adding to the written value of the fixed assets (excluding the surgery) shown in the balance sheet, the total required working capital of the partnership. Figure 18.1 illustrates this; it takes into account the fixed assets (£59 264) together with the stock and debtors, and deducts from these the current liabilities to arrive at £66 895. Added to this figure is the estimated amount the partners require to run the practice on a day-to-day basis for the ensuing month. Most practices receive money on a regular monthly basis and can fairly accurately estimate the amount required to meet all known expenses during a typical month. This figure has been calculated at £13 000. The total figure arrived at by this process is £79 895, rounded up for ease of accounting to £80 000, which will remain constant unless there are significant variations in ensuing years, such as a substantial investment by the partners in fixed assets, which will greatly increase this total.

Fixed capital accounts are also of benefit in arriving at an agreed amount of capital, which can be utilised by the partners when joining or leaving a

	£	£
Fixed assets (at written-down value)		59 264
Current assets:		
Stock	1 275	
Debtors	12 946	
	17 221	
Less: Due to former partner	(948)	
Sundry creditors	(8642)	7 631
		66 895
Cash requirement (on monthly basis)		13 000
Fixed capital requirement		79 895
(rounded)		80 000

Figure 18.1 Calculation of fixed capital requirement at 30 June 1999

practice. If, therefore, in the example given, a partner is to retire with a one-fifth share of the profits, then it would be reasonable for him to withdraw his capital of £16 000 (one-fifth of £80 000). It may well be, of course, that he also has funds held in a current account which will effectively represent his undrawn profits, and these should be considered as a separate entity.

By the same token, such a system of fixed capital can more easily quantify the capital that will be required from a new partner on joining the practice. If, from the example given below, a new partner was to join the practice on an initial share of the profits of, say, 12%, rising to 15% after one year, 18% after two years and then to parity at 20% after three years, his capital contributions would be as follows:

		£
First year 12%		9600
Second year 3%		2400
Third year 3%		2400
Fourth year 2%		1600
		16 000

Having established how the practice's capital can be estimated, use can also be made of this knowledge to so organise the capital on the loans taken out to finance it, in a way which gives the partners the maximum possible tax advantage.

Refinancing surgery loans

In any surgery-owning partnership, a major item of expenditure is the interest on the loan originally taken out on the surgery development. It is normal for such loans to be taken out on a partnership basis, so that the interest is passed through the partnership accounts and effectively relieved for tax. This principle also extends to interest which was 'rolled up' during the period of development before the surgery was occupied. It is essential that the tax relief attracted by this loan is not only properly organised, but is maximised.

GPs can also make use of the present tax law to obtain top rate tax relief on interest paid on a loan taken out to introduce capital into the partnership. By this means, the partnership's surgery loan might be repaid, then taking out individual loans which are injected into the partnership and effectively replace the original borrowing.

Referring to the accounts set out in Chapter 10, the practice owns a surgery at a book value of £631 471, which is secured on a long-term mortgage of £426 426 (*see* Note 21, page 78) with the Branshire Bank plc. Note 20 (page 78) tells us that the property is owned by four partners only, and on page 76 (Note 15) we see that during the year the practice paid £40 264 in loan interest against a charge of £48 697 in the year 30 June 1999, the fall presumably arising from lower interest rates during the second period.

Let us then say that, on 1 July 1999, the partnership repaid that surgery loan by drawing a cheque for the amount outstanding and paying this to the lending bank involved. This entailed a substantial overdrawing on the partnership bank current account for a limited period, which would have required the knowledge and agreement of the bank. At the same time, the four surgery-owning partners agreed with their bank to take out separate loans in their own names for the purpose of introducing capital into the partnership. Provided they maintained that the loan was for this reason, the partners should have had no undue difficulty in obtaining the consequent tax relief. In this case, each of the four partners took out a personal loan of £106 106.50 (a quarter of £424 426).

GPs are taxed on a self-employed basis, under Schedule D, which means that profits earned for, say, the year ended 30 June 1999 will be assessed for tax under the current year basis in the year 1999/2000. By this means, about half of the tax to be earned in that year would be paid during the year of account, with a possible balancing up some months afterwards.

The effect of the introduction of the current year basis of assessment from 1997/98 (see Chapter 22) means that the cash flow benefit has been reduced by about 12 months. Nevertheless, schemes of dividing the surgery loans into the names of the property-owning partners remains attractive for a number of reasons:

- tax relief will be transferred to the actual year basis
- 'double' tax relief will be obtainable for a limited initial period
- where partners wish to make private pension contributions, which depend on the level of profits assessable for the tax year, relevant income upon which pension relief will be granted will be proportionately greater.

Before going ahead with such a scheme, the property-owning partner should, however, be aware of a number of potential problems.

- Care should be taken to ensure that there is no overriding penalty on the redemption of an existing partnership loan. Some lending organisations have tried to impose harsh conditions where such loans are repaid, not only charging penalties but seeking to impose undue restrictions on the personal loans which succeed it.
- An arrangement fee may be charged by the bank for taking out each new loan. In addition, there may be a charge for legal fees, which should be avoided if possible.
- A lending institution will wish to secure the borrowings. As the loans are in the personal names of the individual partners, it will be necessary for cross guarantees to be given so that if, say, a partner dies in service or retires, the bank has the security of knowing that his loan continues to be covered.
- Detailed arrangements should be made to cover the eventuality of partners leaving or retiring from practice. This may necessitate an amendment to the partnership deed.

Tax-efficient borrowing: unlocking the partnership capital

In many practices, the partners have significant sums of capital invested in their partnership, which is effectively of little use to them, apart from financing their investment in the surgery assets and working capital. Given the correct circumstances, it is possible to utilise this capital to replace tax-inefficient borrowing, to attract a higher rate of tax relief than would otherwise be possible and to consolidate personal borrowing into a single source of finance.

Many partners have outstanding loans on which they gain either no tax relief or relief restricted to the basic rate. Such loans may have been those taken out to cover excessive personal spending, or to pay school fees or a house mortgage in excess of £30 000. Overdrafts and borrowings on credit cards are other examples of borrowings which are inefficient for tax purposes.

It is possible to repay these inefficient borrowings and replace them by loans which carry tax relief at the highest rate, as shown in Figure 18.2. This is normally commenced by the partner arranging for his bank to set up a new personal loan account, taken out entirely for the purpose of introducing capital into the partnership. Once this principle has been established, the partner can then draw a cheque on the partnership account up to the amount of his borrowing, and use this to repay loans which do not attract tax relief. He will then draw down the borrowing on the new personal loan arrangement with his bank and use it to replenish his capital account by paying the cheque into the partnership. It is essential that these

Dr Green, who has an agreed level of investment of £17 600 in the fixed capital of his partnership, wishes to refinance this in order to repay borrowings on which no tax relief is being received

	£
Personal overdraft	4000
School fees loan	8000
Credit card borrowings	3500
Loan for house extension (1991)	4500
	20 000

He negotiates with his bank manager a new personal loan of £17 600, for the purpose of introducing capital into the partnership, at an interest rate of 1.5% over base, secured on his share of the partnership capital. He cannot borrow the full £20 000 as this is above the level of his capital balance.

He then draws a cheque for £17 600 on the partnership account, with the agreement of his partners, and uses this to repay the latter three loans (£16 000 in all), with the balance of £1600 being set against his overdraft. The following day he draws the full amount of his new loan, so replenishing the partnership account. This will enable him to receive tax relief as follows:

	£
Interest (pa) on £17 600 at 9.0%	1584
Tax relief at 40%	634

Figure 18.2 How to transfer borrowings to obtain maximum tax relief (based on specimen practice accounts in Chapter 10)

transactions are completed in the correct sequence, and that the bank manager's cooperation is obtained in advance.

This process can be implemented by one or more partners in a practice; other partners who may not wish, or have no need, to participate need not do so.

It must again be strongly emphasised that the extent of the benefit which a partner can obtain by this means is limited to the amount of his capital investment in the practice. This will be apparent from a glance at the practice accounts which will show the amount outstanding on his capital account. There is little point, for instance, in a partner with a capital balance of £5000 seeking to take out a loan of, say, £20 000. This would almost certainly result in the tax relief not being granted and the partner will effectively have lost the cost of fees in setting up the new arrangement, without any consequent benefit. Moreover, the capital account balance should not go below the amount borrowed, or tax relief will again be lost.

Where a partner already has personal borrowings, either in respect of the surgery or other partnership capital, he can still increase his borrowings if there is capital equity remaining. For this purpose, and provided a realistic valuation is used, he must first repay all relevant borrowing and then take out an entirely new loan for the larger amount.

These processes are extremely complex and it is emphasised that they should only be carried out with expert professional advice.

19 Training practices

Some practices are authorised to employ GP registrars during their vocational training period. Only GPs who have undergone a three-year vocational training period are allowed to join practices as principals, and young doctors who propose to enter general practice must therefore comply with these requirements. In this chapter, the financial arrangements that apply to the trainer and registrar are considered.

It is normal for at least one GP in a partnership to be appointed a trainer. In larger partnerships, two or more registrars may be engaged simultaneously, provided the requisite number of partners have been approved as trainers. In financial terms, the trainer receives a supervision grant as recompense for the work involved, while the practice receives reimbursement from the HA for the registrar's salary and other payments made on his behalf.

It is important that the refund received from the HA matches the amount paid to the registrar (*see* Figure 19.1). In legal and taxation terms, the registrar is an employee of the trainer (or of his partnership), who is legally accountable to the Inland Revenue for tax under the PAYE regulations and Class 1 NIC.

	Paid by practice (monthly) £		Recovered from HA £
Recovered from HA: gross salary			2144 (2)
Net salary to registrar (1)		1600	
Paid to Collector of Taxes: PAYE	400 (3)		
Class 1 NIC:			
Employer	166 (4)		166 (4)
Employee	144 (5)	710	
		2310	2310
(1) Net salary calculated (gross):			(2) 2144
Less: Tax (3)		400	
NIC (5)		144	544
			(1) 1600

Figure 19.1 The GP trainee: salary refund August 1999. Figures for illustration purposes only

Some HAs calculate the trainee refund on a quarterly basis; in these cases, the practice should ensure that monthly payments on account are received to maintain good cash flow.

Income tax

The practice should operate PAYE on the employee's salary, including London weighting where appropriate, and any other increments that may apply, including the car allowance and any other amount that might be paid to the registrar above his normal salary.

Income tax need not be applied to refunds of expenditure, such as telephone charges, removal expenses and defence society subscriptions.

National Insurance

The registrar's salary is fully chargeable to Class 1 NIC under the normal rules in force and using tables supplied to the employer. These should be applied at the contracted-out rate (but *see* p. 138) for separate NIC rules applying to the trainee car allowance).

Registrar's superannuation

On the HA remittance statement to the practice, 6% of the registrar's salary is deducted in respect of superannuation contributions. More may be deducted if the registrar is buying added years. The practice must ensure that these deductions are recovered from the registrar's salary before payment, otherwise the trainer and the practice will be out of pocket. Superannuation should be deducted from the gross pay before the PAYE tax is calculated, but it is not deductible when calculating Class 1 NIC.

The supervision grant

The supervision grant is paid to the trainer as part of the remuneration for services as a trainer. This should be allocated in accordance with the wishes of the partners as set out in the partnership deed and displayed in the annual accounts. In some practices this will be retained by the trainer personally; in most cases it will be aggregated with partnership profits for division.

Superannuation at the trainer's own rate (standard plus added years if applicable) is deducted from the supervision grant on payment by the HA, and this should be charged in the partnership current accounts to the trainer concerned, unless election has been made to the HA for it to be allocated in partnership ratios.

Other payments and refunds

Occasionally, various payments will be made to the trainer by way of refund from the HA in respect of payments made by the trainee. These should be passed on to whoever has made the original payment. For instance, payments made in part reimbursement of defence society subscriptions by the registrar should be passed on to him. If reimbursements are made, he can claim tax relief only on the net amount after deduction of the refund.

Removal expenses may well have originally been paid by the registrar and should also be paid over to him. No tax is chargeable if these are genuine reimbursements, and below a statutory threshold. Similarly, with regard to refunds of telephone rentals, if the original bills were paid by the practice then the refund should be paid into the partnership account.

The registrar's car allowance

The car allowance and the means by which it should be taxed cause much controversy.

Under strict tax law, this allowance is part of the registrar's salary; it is paid as part of his contract with the NHS and is properly assessable to income tax. However, provided certain procedures are applied, relief can be obtained for some or all of the amount paid. It is suggested that the following procedure is adopted, in order of preference shown below.

1 The PAYE tax district of the practice should be approached to obtain a general clearance for the car allowance to be paid to the trainee without deduction of tax. If this is accepted by the Inspector of Taxes, the problem is largely solved, for the practice if not for the trainee.

Once obtained, clearance normally applies to successive trainees and will not have to be reapplied for when a new trainee is engaged. The allowance should merely be paid over to the trainee by adding one twelfth of the annual rate of allowance to his salary, there being no need to operate the PAYE system.

Some tax districts are not prepared to give this clearance, and we must then look at the next stage.

2 The registrar should be asked to approach his own tax district (normally the district dealing with the PAYE affairs of the practice) and ask for an increase to his code number to take account of the car allowance. If this is provided, the trainer can operate the PAYE system using the higher coding. This will give the same result as if the clearance outlined above had been granted.

3 If points 1 and 2 are both unacceptable to the tax district, the only alternative is for the trainer, for his own and his practice's protection, to deduct tax from the registrar on the whole of the car allowance as well as his salary, using the code number he is given. It must be emphasised that the negotiation of such a code number is the responsibility of the registrar and not of the employer.

   If this situation applies, it is likely that the trainee can obtain a refund at the end of the year, provided it can be demonstrated clearly to the Inspector of Taxes that the money has been spent on running the car for the use of the practice. This will normally be done using generally accepted principles (*see* Chapter 25).

It is convenient for claims of this nature by GP registrars to be submitted using Inland Revenue form P87.

   It must be emphasised that the responsibility for deducting tax and National Insurance from this car allowance lies with the employer (the trainer). If the Inland Revenue finds that he has not operated tax according to the rules in force, large sums of unpaid tax covering several years could be due from the trainer.

   Registrars should approach their PAYE tax office for local rulings as to the charging of Class 1 NIC on the car allowance.

20 Dispensing practices
Michael Gilbert

A minority of NHS practices are permitted to dispense drugs and appliances to their own patients. This dispensing facility leads to a number of accounting problems.

Generally, in order to qualify as a dispensing practice and be accepted under the scheme, patients for whom the dispensing facility is made available should reside more than one mile from the nearest pharmacist. This usually limits dispensing practices to rural and a few suburban areas: those areas in the UK which have the greatest proportion of dispensing practices are Lincolnshire and North Yorkshire. There is continuing controversy between dispensing doctors and the pharmacists' associations over the right to dispense, as on the one hand GPs' dispensing facilities give a greatly increased level of service to patients, and on the other hand they can deprive qualified pharmacists (who might give a better service) of their livelihood.

Detailed regulations for the calculation of reimbursements to dispensing doctors are contained in paragraph 44 of the SFA. This stipulates that the payments should be calculated under six separate headings.

1 The basic price, calculated in accordance with the group tariff currently in force. From this price an average figure is deducted for estimated discount, which is discussed further below.
2 An oncost allowance of 10.5% of the basic price before the deduction of such a discount.
3 A container allowance of 3.8p per prescription.
4 A dispensing fee, which is on a sliding scale, according to the number of scrips issued per month.
5 An addition in respect of VAT at the rate currently in force.
6 Any exceptional expenses provided for by the drug tariff.

Profitability

Many dispensing practices are highly profitable. The level of profit earned from dispensing depends on the efficiency with which the facility is conducted, and on the following factors.

- The turnover of stock. A quick turnover of drugs means that large amounts of capital are not held up for lengthy periods, although inevitably some drugs become obsolete and may have to be discarded. Some dispensing practices are able to control this by means of a stock control computer program, which allows for reordering when stocks reach a certain level.
- Discounts obtained from pharmaceutical suppliers. The supply of drugs of this nature is highly competitive and there are generally discounts available to practices which can take advantage of them.

On the other hand, partners in a dispensing practice are usually required to contribute a higher level of capital than those in a similar, but non-dispensing, practice. The required stock of drugs, even if kept at a reasonably low level, together with the fact that drug refunds are received up to three months in arrears, means that the current assets of the practice are likely to run at a high level. The high earnings of the partners in part represent a return on this higher investment in the practice capital.

Payments by the HA

Drug refunds to dispensing practices are nearly always made in arrears, sometimes up to three months, although in the majority of cases payments on account are obtained one or two months in arrears. At any given date, such practices therefore carry a substantial amount of capital. They should try to ensure that payments on account are received regularly and at as high a level as can be negotiated, although the partners must accept that carrying relatively high levels of working capital is one of the obligations of running a dispensing practice.

Superannuation

As we have seen, part of the remuneration of the dispensing GP is in the form of a dispensing fee for each scrip submitted. Such dispensing fees are fully superannuable and are subject to deductions at the standard rate of 6%, or higher if any of the doctors are buying added years.

It is essential that superannuation deductions are identified and shown, as with similar deductions from fees and allowances, as part of the charge to each individual doctor through their own current accounts. The practice should ensure that proper elections are submitted to the HA so that these contributions are allocated in partnership ratios.

Stock on hand

At each annual account date, the stock of drugs should be properly valued and shown in the accounts at that value. Many practices employ specialist valuers who come to the surgery shortly after close of business on an account date, to count and check the drugs on hand. These can, if necessary, be valued first and the calculations made at a later date. The stock on hand should include VAT at the rate in force, which would have been paid on these drugs when they were bought. Some practices prefer to have such valuations taken by the doctors and staff, if necessary paying overtime in respect of the additional work entailed.

The valuation should be made on the basis of cost or market value, whichever is the lower. If drugs have been bought at a specially discounted rate, which was less than their true value, it is this rate that should be taken into account when the drugs are valued. Drugs which have no value, or which have been given free by representatives, should not be included in the valuation.

It is essential that this valuation is made and included in the practice accounts. If, as occasionally occurs, a nominal value is included, or worse, the stock is ignored, the profits of the practice will have been understated and the Inland Revenue would be justified in reassessing the tax, possibly for several years in arrears.

Prescribing doctors

GPs in non-dispensing practices can, under SFA Section 44.5, claim a refund and fee under similar arrangements to those outlined above. This normally applies to the supply of vaccines, anaesthetics, injections and family planning devices, etc.

However, if the dispensing practitioner supplies a prescription to a patient, with that patient's consent, rather than supplying the drug from his own dispensary, no remuneration will be paid.

Self-administered drugs

Drugs which were administered by a GP, rather than by a chemist, have previously been held to be exempt from VAT. In a recent VAT tribunal case during 1999, however, it was held that the liability of self-administered drugs to dispensing patients is zero rated, the same as dispensed drugs. Even further, the liability of self-administered drugs supplied to non-dispensing

	1999		1998	
	£	£	£	£
Cost of goods sold				
Stock at 1 July 1998		3940		3228
Purchases during year		37 761		36 174
		41 701		39 402
Less: Stock at 30 June 1998		4275		3940
Cost of drugs dispensed		37 426		35 462
Proceeds:				
Refunds (including VAT, etc.) (Note 10)	49 745		38 877	
Dispensing fees (Note 9)	3462	53 207	2546	41 423
Dispensing profit for the year		15 781		5961
Percentage profit return		29.7%		14.4%

The practice has improved its profitability from its dispensing facility, both in terms of actual profit realised and the percentage return. This may have come about through increased efficiency, improved stock control, a higher discount available, or a combination of all three. Where amounts are received by way of private prescriptions, total income from this source should be included in such a trading account.

The figures are taken from the specimen accounts in Chapter 10, pages 66–81.

Figure 20.1   The trading account of a dispensing practice

patients was held to be standard rated. This confuses even more the situation with regard to the VAT rules for dispensing practices. As we go to press it may well be that Customs and Excise will appeal against this decision, but practices who find themselves in this position should seek up-to-date specialist advice.

Accounting problems

The accounts in Chapter 10 are for a dispensing practice. Figure 20.1 calculates profit earned by that practice over two years.

There are some problems that can arise where accounts are prepared and presented for dispensing practices. None of these are by any means insoluble, given the necessary experience and knowledge to deal with them.

Accounts presentation

Some accountants, when preparing accounts for dispensing practices, will prepare a trading account on the lines set out above, but will merely show as a credit to the income and expenditure account, the dispensing profits for the year (for 1998/99: £15 781). This is wrong; it does not set out the total income and total expenditure of the practice in an acceptable form and effectively is 'netting-out'. This is incorrect and accounts should not be presented in this manner. Failure to do so could well result in the accounts giving incorrect information if selected for the Review Body process. Further, they will not give the information required by the annual partnership income tax return.

Using the illustration above, therefore, there should be shown as an item of income in these accounts the actual refunds and fees received, as separate items, but totalling £53 207. The cost of purchases during the year should be shown at the figure of £37 426. This will give exactly the same result and an identical practice profit as the alternative method but, as has been explained, will give a correct picture to accord with the Review Body requirements. Authority for this treatment is set out in SFA paragraph 44.12.

Provision for debtors

Accounts prepared for GPs are invariably arranged on an income and expenditure basis, which is to say that they record the actual earnings and expenditure of a practice during a given year, rather than amounts actually received and paid, which may well be very different.

Most dispensing practices are paid their drug fees, refunds and similar items several months in arrear. It is by no means unusual to find such fees being paid three months in arrears. Similar arrangements will apply for prescribing practices. It is essential that these are recorded in the accounts of the practice and treated as sundry debtors. This will mean that, where proper accounting has taken place, the accounts as presented will represent the actual amounts earned during the year, rather than those merely received.

Some Inspectors of Taxes offices have raised this with professional advisors and, in a final analysis, practices could find themselves paying heavy arrears of tax if debtors are not properly recorded. This is becoming even more important with the introduction of new rules for the taxation of professional businesses.

Sundry creditors

By exactly the same token, any bills outstanding for drug supplies at the year end will have to be brought into account as sundry creditors. In a large dispensing practice this could run to several thousands of pounds and to ensure the accuracy of the accounts it is essential that the correct procedure be applied.

21 The single-handed practitioner

The majority of GPs in this country practise as members of partnerships. The single-handed practitioner is now in the minority, yet it is a status that retains a few advantages for those who wish to practise in this manner.

Advantages of single-handed practice

The advantages are chiefly related to independence. Some single-handed practitioners have been members of partnerships and either have not relished the experience or find difficulty in working with close colleagues. However, the complexities of modern medical finance and the advantages of forming partnerships are such that the number of single-handed GPs is likely to gradually diminish.

Disadvantages of single-handed practice

Out-of-hours work

Single-handed GPs, particularly in rural areas, find it difficult to obtain assistance with night and other duties. In urban areas, some may join rotas, but for others the use of locums and deputising services is expensive and is likely to become more so following the introduction of differential rates for payment of night duty fees.

Reference and discussion

Many single-handed GPs find that they are remote from their professional colleagues; they do not have the closeness of the members of a successful partnership, and can at times find it difficult to discuss common problems with their peers.

Earnings levels

The need to cover fully the cost of the various services a GP must use, such as telephone, postage, stationery and accountancy, may reduce earnings.

The average single-handed GP has none of the benefits of the pooling of expenses which takes place in a partnership.

At times of sickness and holidays he is obliged to use the services of locums, which may not be necessary even in a medium-sized partnership.

Appointment of a successor

The single-handed GP has no right to appoint a successor, as does a GP in partnership. On retirement, the vacancy will be put up for interview by the LMC and the HA, so that he will have no voice in choosing a successor to cater for his patients. Some single-handed GPs seek to counteract this by taking a partner or assistant for a year or two before retirement, but this is subject to approval by the HA.

Accounts and finance

In terms of book-keeping, the single-handed practitioner should keep records virtually akin to those kept by a partnership, with the exception of calculating drawings and balancing capital accounts. He will, however, still need to have capital invested in his practice, albeit to a somewhat smaller degree.

The single-handed GP should open a practice bank account, into which all medical earnings are paid and from which will be settled all expenses wholly or partially of a business nature. At the end of each month, he can transfer into his private account such sums as appear reasonable, taking into account future known commitments.

If a single-handed GP seeks to develop his own surgery, as some do, he may encounter difficulties in borrowing money due to his non-partnership status.

Single-handed GPs in isolated areas may be able to engage the services of an assistant doctor and receive the associate allowance to partly fund the salary. Such GPs must be in receipt of rural practice payments, or be practising on an island, and either be in receipt of an inducement payment or the practice should be more than 10 miles from the nearest main surgery or district general hospital.

Compliance with legislation

The single-handed GP, who will probably have a very limited staff, is likely to experience difficulty in both keeping up to date and complying with the bureaucracy and all-pervading legislation which is part of the life of any self-employed businessman and employer. Such legislation as the Data

Protection Act, Health and Safety Acts, employment legislation, PAYE and National Insurance and planning regulations take up a great deal of time. Many GPs prefer to spend their time dealing with patients, as they were trained to do, yet single-handed GPs are unable to share responsibility for dealing with legislative issues.

22 Women GPs

In an increasing number of cases, the woman GP is either the breadwinner or the major earner in the family. Female doctors experience many problems in terms of clinical matters and sex discrimination, and also financial and management problems specific to their sex. It is therefore necessary that the woman doctor, particularly one on the point of entering general practice, is aware of these and is able to cater for them as far as possible.

The increasing number of women GPs and the impact that they are having on general practice can be seen from a recent statistic which showed that woman GP principals in England and Wales represent about 35% of all GPs. This would suggest a UK total of about 12 500 out of some 36 000 GPs (1998 Review Body Report: figure for 1996). Taking into account the number of young women doctors currently qualifying, it is evident that the trend will continue to be upwards, and the problems of women GPs are thus likely to magnify over the years.

In conventional society, women not only bear the children but are charged with the responsibility of raising them within the family. It is also normal practice, but by no means universal, in our society that women are the members of the family unit invariably charged with the routine tasks of catering for the family household and ensuring that it runs in as smooth and efficient a manner as possible. Hence the problems and prejudices that affect working women.

Job sharing

One of the more novel aspects of the 1990 GP contract was its introduction of 'job sharing' as a legally recognised option, particularly to cater for the aspirations of female doctors who cannot devote the whole of their lives and working hours to their practice.

A further variation of the job-sharing facility is the manner in which it has been extended to husband and wife GP teams in a more flexible form. While unrelated job sharers are likely to allocate their minimum 26 hours per week more or less equally, a husband and wife may choose instead for one partner, say the husband, to work 20 hours and his wife six; this is quite acceptable as long as the contract is fulfilled and the practice works in an efficient manner. Such a situation may be compared favourably with the position of other part-time practitioners who are required to work at least 13 hours a week in order to qualify for the BPA.

Maternity allowance

A female employee is entitled to certain protection with regard to maternity leave and her job must be kept open during her absence. However, this does not apply to female GPs, who are not employees but independent contractors and self-employed. They can nevertheless claim certain allowances under the terms of this contract with the NHS.

Detailed conditions for payment of the maternity allowance to female GPs (referred to as additional payments during confinement) are set out in paragraph 49 of the SFA. Generally, the scheme operates on a similar basis to payment during absence through sickness, although there is now no restriction in respect of minimum list sizes.

Payments under the maternity scheme are made to any GP on the medical list, provided she expresses an intention to continue in general practice. They are intended to reimburse her wholly, or partly, for the cost of an external locum whom she has engaged to give clinical care to patients during her absence. Where the doctor in question is a part-time practitioner or job sharer, payments are scaled down accordingly.

Payments will normally continue for a period of 13 weeks maximum, or until such time as the GP re-enters practice. If it is necessary for the practitioner to be away from her practice for longer than 13 weeks due to ill health, she may be able to claim payments under the sickness scheme, although she cannot benefit from both the sickness and maternity schemes simultaneously.

It is essential that the practitioner who either is, or anticipates finding herself, absent from the practice through childbirth, agrees with her partners the exact financial conditions which are to apply and that these are set down in a proper partnership deed.

Partnership deeds

It is essential that a female GP, preferably on joining a practice, agrees with her partners the exact financial provisions which are to apply in the event of any future absence on maternity leave.

There are two main variations which can apply, and a choice will be made according to the policy of the partnership.

- The female GP pays the locums herself during the entire period of her absence and retains the maternity allowance during the 13-week period, or whatever period is covered.
- All transactions are passed through the partnership, which pays the locum fees and retains the maternity allowance.

Under the first of these options, any shortfall in cost is automatically borne by the absent GP, while in the second case any shortfall is covered by the partnership.

For practical reasons, it is better if the locum is physically paid by the female GP out of her own funds and the maternity allowance paid to her on receipt. This avoids confusion where GPs are absent for more than 13 weeks, but the allowance is limited to that length of time. The payment of locums in such circumstances is best kept outside the partnership accounts, as when the accountant comes to draw them up, up to a year later, it may be forgotten which locum fees apply to the maternity period.

Child minding

Female GPs are unable to obtain tax relief for the cost of engaging people to look after their children while they are at work. The case is often made that most women GPs would not be able to work without such a facility and that it is a legitimate charge against tax. Unfortunately, such logic is lost on the Inland Revenue, which consistently declines to accept any such claims. In recent years, some relief has been granted where an employer provides a creche or similar facility for the children of its employees, but this is not extended to self-employed GPs.

Salaries for husbands

Chapter 28 (p. 187) addresses the issue of female doctors paying a salary to their husbands for assistance in their practice. Such a payment is permitted, although it is likely to be less tax efficient than the reverse situation of a husband paying a salary to his wife for assistance in the practice. Payments to older children for similar duties are also discussed on page 189.

Wives' pension schemes

In the case of a female GP who is the wife of a male GP, then it is more likely that the claim will be accepted, as the woman's professional qualification obviously gives her a great deal of value in assisting her husband.

In such circumstances, and particularly if the woman GP has no other source of income, it is essential that the husband pays employee pension premiums on her salary. This, it is suggested, should be an investment priority for the family.

Widowers' pensions

Since 6 April 1988, contributions made by female GPs to the NHS Pension Scheme (NHSPS) have also contributed to the purchase of a pension for the widower in the event of the woman's death either during service or in retirement. Until 30 June 1989, it was possible for female GPs to buy benefit arrears, but this is no longer available and any contributions made will only count towards a widower's pension from 1988. Female doctors who feel that they have not made adequate pension provision should consider the various private pension schemes which are now available (see Chapters 32 and 33).

Surgery ownership

Many female GPs, on entering a practice, do not take part in the acquisition of a share in the surgery building, possibly due to the uncertain duration of their stake in the partnership; for example, they may at some time be required to move location as a result of their husband's employment, or for another reason.

This decision can only be made by the practitioner concerned, in consultation with her partners. However, despite problems with negative equity, ownership of surgeries is an excellent long-term investment, and GPs who decline the opportunity to take part in ownership may well be losing not only a valuable continuing source of income but also a significant capital sum on retirement. Women GPs who anticipate remaining with the practice for a lengthy period should seriously consider buying into the surgery.

Where the GP does not take on the responsibility of surgery ownership, and will not share in any proceeds of the cost or notional rent reimbursement, she should ensure that she is not required to pay any share of interest or repayments on the surgery mortgage, or to pay rent to her partners for the privilege of practising from the surgery.

23 Taxation in general practice

For God's sake madam, don't say that in England, for if you do they will surely tax it.

Jonathan Swift

Taxation of some kind has always been with us and presumably will remain. It comes in several forms: taxes on income, on capital, on the estates of deceased persons and value-added tax (VAT) levied on goods and services. A GP is likely to come across most, if not all, of those forms of taxation during his working life.

The purpose of these chapters is to explain, particularly to new GPs, the principles that apply and the manner in which income from their practices is taxed. Taxation of all types is extremely complex and GPs are well advised to engage the services of a qualified, experienced and specialist accountant to give advice on all aspects of tax. Once an accountant has been employed, the GP should *not* negotiate and correspond separately with the local tax office.

Each year, normally in March, the Chancellor of the Exchequer presents to Parliament a Budget statement, which ultimately becomes the Finance Act for that year. It is rare – but by no means unknown – for proposed legislation to be changed between the announcement of the Budget and the eventual passing of that year's Finance Act into law.

From time to time, the various regulations and statutes are codified in an omnibus act, the latest of these being the Income and Corporation Taxes Act, 1988.

The whole taxation system has been changed in recent years, so far as this affects GPs and other self-employed people. The change to current-year basis (see below) and the new self-assessment procedures (*see* Chapters 23 and 24) have changed radically and for ever the manner in which our tax is assessed and paid.

The Inland Revenue offices

As far as the GP is concerned, the Revenue service is divided into two sections: the Inspector and the Collector. It is the Inspector of Taxes office (now at times referred to by different names, such as 'Taxpayer Service Office') to which annual income tax returns will be submitted and with which the taxpayer, or his agent, will negotiate concerning his tax liability. This office will also, if appropriate, issue penalty notices, interest charges and the like (*see* Chapter 24). The office is staffed by revenue officials of various grades who each have their separate function to perform.

The Collector of Taxes offices throughout the country are responsible for the demand and collection of tax. It is this office to which a tax bill is paid, and which deals with the issue of receipts and takes enforcement proceedings if the tax is not paid.

The various schedules

Income tax is divided into several schedules, each of which governs the rules for assessment of tax on incomes of various types. The schedules currently in force are set out in Box 23.1.

Box 23.1: Income tax: the various schedules

Schedule A: income from property

Schedule B: woodlands

Schedule C: paying agents

Schedule D: Cases I and II: profits from trades, professions, etc.

              Case III: interest receivable

              Cases IV and V: overseas income

              Cases VI: miscellaneous income

Schedule E: earnings from employment: salaries, wages, etc.

Schedule F: dividends, etc.

Employment and self-employment: Schedules D and E

For most GPs, the tax on their incomes will be of greatest concern, and Schedules D and E will be most relevant. The main characteristics of each schedule are set out in Box 23.2.

Box 23.2: Income tax: Schedules D and E

Schedule D

- paid by self-employed (including GPs)
- assessed on current-year basis
- payable twice a year
- more relaxed treatment of expense claims (but *see* Chapter 26 on the detailed preparation of these claims)
- National Insurance: classes 2 and 4 (*see* Chapter 29)

Schedule E

- paid by employees (practice staff, GP trainees, hospital doctors, etc.)
- assessed on actual year basis, and paid over monthly
- payable by deduction from wages/salaries. Stringent treatment of claims for expenses
- National Insurance: class 1 (*see* Chapter 29)

Most GPs at some time will have been assessed for tax under Schedule E and have had deductions made from their salaries under PAYE; they may have been employees of a hospital authority, GP registrars or in other forms of employment.

The GP as a self-employed practitioner is assessed under Schedule D, which derives entirely from his status as an independent contractor.

As the method of assessment in each schedule is different, it is important to understand how these schedules work. The main differences lie in the manner in which expenses are allowed, the basis of assessment and the dates of payment of tax. These rules apply to *all* self-employed taxpayers. The taxation problems arising in medical partnerships are discussed more fully in Chapter 25, while personal expenses claims are dealt with in Chapter 26.

In many cases, these two schedules overlap, with some GPs receiving income simultaneously under both headings. Where this occurs in partnerships, extremely complex situations can arise, and these are discussed more fully in Chapter 25.

Moreover, in many cases, it is not immediately apparent whether the income from any particular appointment is to be assessed under Schedule D or Schedule E. In recent years, the Inland Revenue has examined several professions outside the medical world and redesignated them as Schedule E from Schedule D.

In the medical field, confusion can frequently arise in the treatment of fees paid to locums or assistant GPs. Where fees are paid from practice funds, the proper taxation formalities should be observed. For instance, if a practice engages a doctor at a salary of £15 000 a year and then proceeds to pay that doctor monthly, this constitutes a salary and must be taxed under PAYE. On the other hand, if occasional locum fees are paid to different doctors, calculated on a sessional basis without any true employer–employee relationship, then it is likely that they can be treated as Schedule D income and the recipient must accept the obligation of returning these to the Inland Revenue and paying tax on them.

Years of assessment

Tax is organised on a basis of tax years, sometimes termed 'years of assessment' or 'fiscal years'. In all cases, these years run from 6 April in one calendar year to 5 April in the next. Thus, the year from 6 April 1997 to 5 April 1999 would be designated 1998/99, and that from 6 April 1999 to 5 April 2000 as 1999/2000.

The basis of assessment

A major benefit from Schedule D status is the facility for paying tax twice a year, rather than having it deducted from a weekly or monthly wage or salary, as would apply with employees. This situation arises from the current-year basis of assessment, where profits charged to tax in any year of assessment are based on the profits earned in the accounting period ended within the same tax year. This is known as the current-year basis of assessment.

Up to 1995/96, all tax under Schedule D was assessed on the preceding-year basis, which is to say that profits earned in an accounting year ended, say, 30 June 1994 would be assessed in the tax year 1995/96. That was the last year to which the preceding-year basis applied, the result of which has meant that the tax payable by a Schedule D taxpayer has in effect been brought forward by one year.

1997/98 was the first year in which the current-year basis of assessment comes fully into force. For a practice making up its accounts to any period ending between 6 April 1997 and 5 April 1998 therefore, the tax will be assessed for tax purposes in the fiscal year 1997/98. Practices making up their accounts to 30 June 1998 or 31 March 1999, which are the most common dates to which GP accounts are prepared, will have the tax on those years' profits assessed in 1998/99.

In the following year, accounts made up to 30 June 1999 and 31 March 2000 will be assessed in the tax year 1999/2000.

The transitional year

It follows that, if 1995/96 was the last year to which the preceding-year basis of assessment applies and 1997/98 is the first year to which the current-year basis applies, then there is one year – 1996/97 – missing, but two years of accounts not otherwise assessed. If no adjustment were to be made, then the taxpayer would have found himself paying tax on two years' profits in one year.

This, however, was not the case and the profits for those two years were effectively averaged out to give a single year's assessment.

Example
Dr John makes up his accounts to 30 June annually. His profits for the two years during the transitional period were as follows:

	£
Year ended 30 June 1995	50 000
Year ended 30 June 1996	60 000

Dr John would have been assessed in the 1996/97 year on an amount of £55 000, being the average of those two years.

Dates of payment of tax

With the introduction of the current-year basis and self-assessment, the dates for payment of tax have been altered slightly. Tax is now payable on 31 January and 31 July in each year.

A major problem with the old preceding-year basis of assessment was the complex system for paying income tax and CGT. In many cases, partners who had trading income and investment income would receive numerous assessments with differing dates for payment. Under the new system there are common payment dates for all taxes.

The new current-year basis involves a partner making payments on account in advance of the due date. Generally speaking, a GP will make two equal payments on account, one on 31 January in the tax year and the other one on the following 31 July. These are merely payments on account; if the ultimate tax liability proves to be higher then this must be paid with the following payment following the end of the tax year. The amount of each payment on account will be one half of the GP's total tax liability for the previous year. Conversely, if the liability should prove to be lower than the amounts paid on account, then a refund will be paid.

Example
Dr Peter had a total tax liability for the 1998/99 year of £20 000. When his return is submitted it is found that his liability for the 1999/2000 year is £25 000. For 1999/2000 he will make two payments on accounts, as follows:

		£
31 January 2000		10 000
31 July 2000		10 000
Balancing payment		
31 July 2001		5000
		25 000

It follows that on 31 January 2001 also, he will be required to make his first payment on account of the 2000/2001 liability, which will be £12 500 (one half of £25 000).

Where, as sometimes occurs in GP practices, the profits are found to have risen sharply, then the 31 January liability could well be substantial.

Organisation of accounting date

Under the preceding-year basis, it was fairly conventional advice to propose to GP practices to make their accounts up to 30 June annually. This had two benefits:

* it greatly deferred the date at which tax was payable on a single year's profits
* it coincided with a normal quarter date for NHS fees and allowances.

Under the new system, however, different parameters have come into play. Under the current-year basis of assessment, a major principle is that an individual will be taxed on profits made throughout his career, without any effect of overlapping at either end of the scale. It follows that where a new business commences, some of the profit will be taxed in separate years. The Revenue has granted a system of 'overlap relief', which means that at the end of the GP's career this relief will be allowed against his final year's assessment.

A similar situation will arise on the change to current-year basis, where GPs will have found themselves taxed twice on profits earned in the same period. Again, this will be allowed in a similar manner, being known as 'transitional overlap relief'. Unfortunately, in granting this relief there is no hedge against inflation and when a young doctor of today retires in, say, 30 years' time, the loss in value of money could well mean that this relief is of relatively little value.

The only manner in which this can be avoided is to change the accounting year-end of the practice to 31 March, and many advisors have proposed that this be done. It is, however, not to be embarked upon without a great deal of consideration as there are times when there can be a financial disadvantage to the practice. There are again two factors that come into play.

- The change of a year-end to 31 March will result in overlap relief being granted immediately, when it is of greater value, rather than when it has been subject to inflationary factors over a lengthy period. It will also ultimately result in a partner not having to accept a significantly higher tax liability on his eventual retirement.
- On the other hand, there is less time for the accounts to be produced and partnership tax returns to be submitted. In many cases, a ten-month period (1 April to 31 January) has proved to be exacting, particularly where delays have come about in preparing and completing accounts.

Many practices could well benefit from a change of accounting year-end. It should not, however, be embarked upon without serious consideration and knowledgeable professional advice.

24 Personal taxation

In a publication of this nature, only the most basic of tax rules can be considered. GPs who seek wider knowledge of tax laws as they affect individual taxpayers, should undertake more extensive reading. However, most GPs engage an accountant (*see* Chapter 34) to deal with taxes for them.

The introduction, effectively from 1996/97, of self-assessment for personal taxpayers has revolutionised both the administration and collection of income tax. This is outlined in brief terms below.

Personal allowances

Every UK citizen is entitled to a personal allowance to set against his tax liability for a given year. The system of independent taxation for spouses, introduced in the early 1990s, means that married couples are now assessed separately for tax purposes, each of them being entitled to their own personal allowance.

For 1999/2000, the personal allowance for individuals is £4195. A married couple who individually have income above that level therefore will between them be able to claim a total of £8390 against their combined tax liabilities.

Married couples can also claim an additional married couples' allowance, which is no longer granted in terms of an allowance, but having regard to a tax rate announced from year to year. For 1999/2000, the maximum amount in cash terms of this married couples' allowance is £285. This is interchangeable between husband and wife but will normally be granted to a husband unless an election is made otherwise.

There is no longer any specific tax relief for dependent children, although single-parent families may claim the additional personal allowance, which is identical with the married couples' allowance of £285.

Income tax rates

A gradual reduction in the basic rate of tax has seen this fall twice in recent years, so that for 1999/2000, the rate will be maintained at 23%. There is, however, a lower rate of 10% on the first £1500 of income, with a higher rate band of 40% coming into force when net taxable incomes exceed £28 000.

Payment of tax

We have seen the process by which tax is collected in respect of individual Schedule D taxpayers. Chapter 25 looks at the position with regard to partnerships.

For those who are employees, i.e. GP registrars, hospital doctors, consultants, etc., the majority of their tax will be deducted from their salary under the PAYE system. However, for those with other sources of income, notably from investments, proceeds from private fees and the like, it will be necessary to complete a self-assessment tax return each year and to clear the amount of tax on or before the due date.

Mortgage interest relief

GPs with private mortgages on their own houses will be able to claim tax relief on the interest charge, but only up to a ceiling of £30 000. In recent years there has been a trend towards reducing the effect of tax relief on house mortgages and for 1999/2000, this has been reduced to 10% of interest on a loan up to £30 000.

Interest on mortgages above that level does not normally qualify for relief, although in some cases where GPs can prove that they use their homes for practice purposes, it might be possible to negotiate additional relief.

The MIRAS (Mortgage Interest Relief at Source) system means that such relief is invariably granted at the time the payment is made, by deduction from the interest payment to the bank or building society, and has no effect on the overall tax assessment of the doctor concerned.

Self-assessment

Self-assessment for personal taxpayers, which first applied in 1996/97, has brought with it an entirely new tax regime, involving required dates for submission of returns and a penalty regime where returns are not submitted and/or tax not paid on time.

Self-assessment is a highly complex subject which cannot be covered adequately in this chapter and readers are advised either to seek professional advice or to supplement their knowledge of the matter through specialist literature.

Submission of returns

Self-assessment returns must be submitted by one of two dates. If the taxpayer wishes the Revenue to work out his tax liability for him, then the return must be submitted by the 30 September following the year of assessment. Therefore, a return for the year ended 5 April 2000 must be submitted by 30 September 2000 if this is to apply.

The final date for submission of those returns, however, is the end of January following the end of the year of assessment. If returns are not submitted by that date an automatic fine of £100 applies, with further escalating penalties and interest being applied the longer the return remains outstanding.

Income to be included on self-assessment tax returns will include all income and capital gains of the taxpayer, from whatever source. The taxpayer (or his agent) will work out his tax liability and the amount must then be paid so as to reach the tax office by 31 January at the latest.

Specialist reading

Readers who wish to advance their knowledge of taxation in general for GPs are advised to consult the tax guidance notes issued by the British Medical Association. These cover several topics and are an invaluable guide to taxation for all doctors. Details can be obtained from BMA House.

Although written primarily for accountants, the Institute of Chartered Accountants through Accountancy Books (020 7833 3291) publishes a volume, *Doctors*, which includes valuable advice on taxation. In addition, the same body publishes a series of briefing notes which are updated regularly and give extensive guidance on taxation for GPs.

25 Partnership taxation

We have looked at the taxation system in general practice (Chapter 23) and how this is applied to individuals (Chapter 24).

Perhaps in no other way has the introduction of self-assessment for tax purposes affected individuals as it has done for doctors in partnership. No longer will they be assessed as members of a partnership; the last partnership assessments were issued for the 1996/97 year. In future all partners will be assessed as private individuals, which again has a spin-off effect in other areas.

Change to self-assessment

The chief areas in which GP partners have been affected by the change to self-assessment are as follows.

- Partners are no longer jointly and severally liable for the tax liabilities of their partners. In other words, if a partner defaults on his tax liability, this is a matter between that partner and the Inland Revenue. His partners cannot be held liable for any shortfall. This could well affect the logic of maintaining a tax reserve accounts.
- Many GPs joining partnerships will at some time have signed a continuation election under the old rules. This is no longer relevant and no such elections are required to be signed after 5 April 1997.
- Partnerships are required to complete and submit a detailed income tax return (see below).
- Partnership profits are divided for tax purposes between the partners on the basis of the profit-sharing ratios during the basis period, not those applying during the year of assessment. Under the old system, if a partnership realised profits of, say, £200 000 in the year ended 30 June 1994, these would be assessed in the 1995/96 tax year and would have been divisible between the partners using ratios applicable between 6 April 1995 and 5 April 1996. This system has now ceased and from 1997/98, partners will be personally assessable, but on the basis of profits earned during the accounting year in which the profits were earned.

Types of partner

A business partnership is correctly defined as 'the relationship which exists between persons carrying on business in common with a view to profit'. The less legally minded have been known to refer to a partnership as 'the most intimate form of association outside marriage'.

In general practice there are a number of types of partners, who may well exist side by side in the same practice.

The majority of GPs will be full-time equity partners in their practice, sharing profits in a predetermined ratio. Their earnings in a given year will be their profit-sharing ratio applied to their total partnership profit, after making due allowance for prior charges, such as seniority, PGEA, net surgery income and the like.

Example
Dr Jones is a member of a five-doctor partnership, with a 22% share of the profits. In the year ended 30 June 1998 his partnership earned a total of £220 000, including £20 000 in respect of prior shares. Dr Jones's share of these seniority, PGEA, etc. awards was £4500. His profits were allocated as follows:

	£
£200 000 (£220 000 less £20 000) × 22%	44 000
Add seniority, PGEA, etc.	4500
	48 500

In the 1998/99 tax year, Dr Jones was assessed on £48 500, less such personal expenses (*see* Chapter 26) as he is able to claim.

Fixed-share partners

Some partners will at times be introduced on the basis of a fixed share of the profits. In the example quoted above, if Dr Jones's share of the profits had been, say, £30 000, then his profit for the year would be £30 000 plus prior charges £4500 = £34 500.

It must be emphasised that for taxation purposes these doctors are partners in every sense of the word; the criterion as to whether a doctor is a partner or not is whether or not he receives the BPA. When accounts are drawn up, the income paid to those doctors should be in the form of an appropriation of profit, rather than a charge as a 'salary' in the income and expenditure account. Under no circumstances whatever should these doctors be referred to as 'salaried partners'. The term 'fixed-share partner' says much the same thing but there are less potential taxation disadvantages.

It must be emphasised that a doctor working on a regular basis in a practice can be one of two things; either he is a partner or an employee. If he does not receive the BPA, then he must be treated as an employee in every sense of the word, with PAYE/NIC being applied to his salary. There is no halfway house; a doctor engaged on a permanent basis cannot be treated as some sort of 'self-employed locum'. He is an employee in every sense of the word and must be treated as such.

Schedule E remuneration in partnerships

Until very recently this was a topic that caused a great deal of conflict, often with tax offices but occasionally between partners. This arose where the Inland Revenue insisted on taxing the partner in whose name the appointment was held on the income earned from such an appointment, despite the fact that it was paid into his partnership account and shared between the partners.

Fortunately this situation has now been resolved and doctors finding themselves in this position should without undue difficulty be able to negotiate an NT coding for this income, provided the amount received is small in comparison with the totality of partnership income, which is invariably the case.

Where such tax deductions continue it is suggested that the doctor or his accountant contacts the tax office immediately, to ensure that an NT coding is issued. It must be emphasised that this regulation applies to doctors in partnership and not to sole practitioners.

The partnership tax return

With the new self-assessment regime has come a requirement that all partnerships will be required to submit a partnership tax return. The first of these returns to be submitted under the new rules was for the 1996/97 year. The return will normally be required to be signed by a representative partner, normally the senior or finance partner. This return must show all the partners who have been in the practice during the period covered, their names, home addresses, tax reference and National Insurance numbers.

In the return is a page showing expenditure of the partnership as a whole, in this figure must be included all the partners' personal expenses to be claimed (see Chapter 26). If they are not included in this total figure on the partnership return, the claim will be lost.

As with individuals, there is a deadline for submission of the return, which is 31 January following the end of the tax year. A return for the 1999/2000 tax year must therefore be submitted at the latest by 31 January

2001. If the return is not submitted on time there is a fixed penalty of £100 for each partner, together with a further penalty of £100 if each partner has still not been submitted after the filing date. There are provisions for even more stringent penalties in certain circumstances.

Personal practice expenses

The manner in which doctors are able to claim expenses incurred privately against their own share of the partnership income tax assessment is discussed more fully in Chapter 26. Each partner will submit, or have prepared for him by his accountant, an annual claim for personal practice expenses which is allowable against tax in exactly the same manner as partnership profits are assessed, i.e. on the preceding-year basis.

Therefore, if five GPs are in a partnership making up its annual accounts to 30 June, each of them will prepare a practice expenses claim made up to 30 June annually. GPs are not employees and should not prepare expenses claims up to a 5 April year-end unless this happens to coincide with the annual accounting date of the partnership.

These expenses, once formulated and agreed with the Inland Revenue, will be allowed for tax against that partner's share of the profits and no other. In large partnerships these expenses claims can vary widely as partners' personal circumstances may differ considerably. This will inevitably affect their own share of the partnership tax liability.

Interest received

Some partnerships will receive interest on deposit accounts or funds held in building societies and this will normally be paid after the deduction of tax.

This income is not assessable with the remainder of the Schedule D trading profits of the partnership, but will be taken out outside that assessment and will be charged individually to the partners in the proportions in which they have received it. It is usual for those amounts to be entered separately in the personal tax returns of each partner but they must also be shown on the partnership return.

The property-owning partnership

The shares of ownership frequently differ from those in which practice profits are shared.

It is necessary in such circumstances to exclude transactions applying to the surgery ownership from the initial allocation for tax purposes, bringing them in at a later stage but dividing the net profit or loss accruing in the shares in which the building is owned during the year of assessment. See also Chapter 15.

Further reading

For further and more detailed information about partnership taxation, the reader is referred to the successive annual issues of *Tolley's Tax Planning*, by the same author, which includes a detailed chapter on various aspects of partnership taxation for GPs.

26 Personal expenses
Michael Gilbert

There are few areas that cause such controversy as the extent and manner in which the GP claims tax relief in respect of expenses paid privately, but which wholly or partly involve practice use. It is an area likely to bring the GP into dispute with his accountant and, possibly, the Inland Revenue.

The attitude of the Inland Revenue has changed considerably in recent years; overclaiming of personal expenses by GPs can have serious consequences.

Partnership or personal expenses?

Most of the expenditure met by a GP or, more likely, his partnership, is of a routine nature and not likely to be disputed by the Inland Revenue, e.g. printing and stationery, surgery telephone bills, staff wages and locum fees.

The categories of expenditure paid personally vary from one partnership to another. The policy of the partners will determine what expenditure is paid out of partnership funds and what is paid privately. Whatever the policy, it should be mutually agreed and set down in the partnership deed. It is important for an incoming partner to determine exactly which expenses have to be met personally.

The major items of expenditure likely to be paid personally by the partners are set out in Box 26.1. Of these, spouses' salaries (*see* Chapter 28) and motor expenses (*see* Chapter 27) are dealt with later.

Box 26.1: Practice expenses: items likely to be paid personally

- house expenses
- motor expenses
- spouse's salary, pension, etc.
- defence society and other medical subscriptions
- private telephone bills
- personal locum fees
- educational course fees and conferences
- locum cover insurance premiums

The basic rule

The basic rule applicable to the claiming of personal expenses, for Schedule D purposes, is that they must be seen by the Inland Revenue as having been expended wholly and exclusively for the purpose of the profession.

Thus, the GP who pays locum fees to another doctor for covering his out-of-hours duties is allowed those fees for income tax purposes. If he were an employed doctor, it is highly unlikely that the expense would be allowed because the additional qualifying word in the case of Schedule E expenses, 'necessarily', might be impossible to justify.

Claims for personal practice expenses in respect of GPs in partnership should always be made up to the same date as the practice's accounting year-end, even if a GP joined midway through the year. Thus, if Dr E joined the partnership on 1 February 1998 and the partnership makes up its accounts to 30 June annually, Dr E's first claim should be for the five-month period to 30 June 1998, and to that same annual date in succeeding years.

Of far greater difficulty are those expenses which the GP pays partially for private and partially for practice use – for instance, a private car or telephone used partly for practice purposes. In fractional terms, the appropriate amount to claim must be based on the facts of each individual case.

A further concept the Inland Revenue applies is 'duality of purpose'. What this means is that if expenditure is incurred simultaneously both for private and practice use, the expenditure will be wholly disallowable. This is subject to a number of interpretations, most of which the average taxpayer may consider to be 'splitting hairs'. Thus, a GP who buys suits to use in his consulting room would be unable to obtain any tax relief for that expenditure because the Revenue considers suits to be primarily for a private purpose with some incidental element of practice use. On the other hand, the same principle is unlikely to be applied to such expenses as motoring costs, the Inland Revenue fully accepting an agreed element of practice use as allowable.

The attitude of the Inland Revenue

Historically, GPs have received relatively generous treatment from the Inland Revenue in the scrutiny of their expenses claims. However, there has been a change of approach in recent years. There is some evidence that the accounts and claims of self-employed GPs, both medical and dental, have been subject to particularly close examination and that Inspectors of Taxes have queried such claims under a number of headings.

Experience has shown that claims for salaries paid to spouses, motor expenses, practice use of houses and telephone costs are particularly vulnerable. The inclusion of estimates is also penalised in some cases. It is in the power of the Inland Revenue to investigate past tax years, and this new, more stringent, attitude has been very costly for a few unfortunate GPs.

Where the Inland Revenue is able to establish a pattern of overclaiming lasting for several years, it is empowered to increase assessments retrospectively, possibly over as much as six years, seeking to collect not only lost tax, but also interest and penalties. It is essential that GPs making claims for expenses, and discussing with their accountants the manner in which these are formulated, should understand the risk of unrealistic claims instigating an in-depth investigation. In particular, it should be ensured that:

- all claims submitted are clearly justified and that the expenditure has been made for practice purposes
- receipts are available to support all claims
- where restrictions for private use are in force, they can be justified
- claims showing estimated expenditure are avoided so far as is possible. Where these are unavoidable, the fact that they are estimates should be clearly shown on the claims submitted to the Inland Revenue.

GPs should understand that, when a claim is prepared on their behalf by an accountant, the onus is on them to keep the accountant informed of genuine expenses incurred *and* to check draft claims before submission to ensure that no unjustified or incorrect claims are made. The GP should be asked to sign the claim as correct before it is submitted to the Inland Revenue.

What can be claimed?

Claims can fall under a number of general headings.

- Expenditure paid personally by the GP but which can clearly be demonstrated as being solely for practice purposes, such as medical equipment, medical journals and subscriptions.
- Expenses incurred for partially practice and partially private use, such as home telephone and motoring.
- Expenses for which the GP wishes to claim but can produce no receipts or invoices, and estimates, may be submitted. However, as has been outlined above, claims of this nature are particularly at risk of attracting unwanted Revenue attention.

GPs frequently ask 'What claims am I entitled to make?' In short, they have no entitlement to claim anything; indeed claiming an expense and having it allowed by the Revenue are two separate matters. A GP can look for ever at the Income Tax Acts and will find no reference to doctors' cars, houses and the like. Overclaiming on expenditure and hoping that the Inland Revenue will allow it is unprofessional and the penalties for overclaiming can be serious.

The preparation of such claims can cause dissent between the GP and the accountant. An accountant who advises his client to moderate claims to a level which will be acceptable to the Inland Revenue, yet which do not deprive the GP of any tax relief to which he might legitimately be due, is attempting to protect his client in advance from an Inland Revenue enquiry. The accountant is acting in the long-term interests of the GP, and the latter should accept advice of this nature.

How are personal expenses claimed?

Following the introduction of self-assessment on 6 April 1996, it is now essential that claims for personal expenses are incorporated within self-assessment Income Tax Returns.

In the case of a sole practitioner, his personal expenses will be incorporated within his annual accounts. These will then be further included within his or her self-assessment Income Tax Return.

As regards partners, their individual personal expenses can be incorporated within the main body of the partnership accounts, which will then be included within the Partnership Tax Return. Alternatively, where the personal expenses are not incorporated with the partnership accounts they must still be amalgamated with the partnership expenses and duly declared as the Partnership Tax Return.

Once the Partnership Tax Return has been completed, the partners are advised of their individual shares of profit to be declared on their own self-assessment Income Tax Returns. These shares of profit are thus net of personal expenses.

Practice use of home

The majority of GPs use their home to a greater or lesser degree for practice purposes. Some GPs have no central surgery, and some single-handed practitioners have a surgery in part of their house. Such doctors have a legitimate claim for a share of the costs of running the house. At the other end of the scale, GPs living several miles away from the practice area, who use their homes mainly for occasional study or reference purposes, cannot make claims on the same basis.

Proportions of house expenses

Claims are frequently made for practice use of GPs' houses, based on the proportion which the practice use of the house bears to the total floor area, or by some similar means. Such claims, possibly when extended to include qualifying repairs expenditure and excess mortgage interest, can be substantial.

To ensure that such claims are justified, they should be made only when:

- there is clear evidence of the use of the house for consulting or treatment of patients on a regular basis
- a professional plate is displayed outside the house (although not mandatory, this could make the acceptance of a borderline claim more likely)
- there is an appropriate entry in the local telephone directory
- the house is either within, or adjacent to, the practice area.

If the claim is to be fully justified, the first point must apply.

Having established that the basis for such a claim exists, it is necessary to calculate the fractional cost of the total house expenses to be claimed. The method usually employed, and which is invariably acceptable to the Inland Revenue, is to award an arbitrary points figure to every room in the house, more or less dependent on its size, and then to allocate those points between practice and private use (*see* Figure 26.1). For instance, if there is a study where patients are seen and which is used for no other purpose, all of the points attributable to this room can be allocated to practice use. Conversely, it is unlikely that an upstairs bedroom or bathroom can be allocated other than wholly for private use. This system may be based on floor areas, but this may be felt to be overcomplication.

The expenses included in the claim should be the normal running costs of the house, *excluding* capital expenditure.

Figure 26.2 shows a worked example of a typical claim for a GP's house expenses, with none of the rooms used exclusively for practice use, but which finally gives a fractional figure of one-seventh to be claimed. Although the principle of this method is likely to be acceptable to an Inspector of Taxes, the allocation of the various rooms may be negotiable.

Dr B Truman, 'Watneys', 19 Courage Road, Worthington-on-Bass

	Practice	Private	Total
Downstairs:			
Garage (double)	12	8	20
Kitchen	1	14	15
Lounge (waiting)	2	18	20
Dining room	–	15	15
Study (consulting)	7	3	10
Entrance hall	1	4	5
Cloakroom	1	4	5
Storage room	1	4	5
Upstairs:			
Main bedroom	–	20	20
3 bedrooms (15 each)	–	45	45
Bathroom	–	10	10
WC	–	5	5
	25	150	175

Figure 26.1   Practice proportion of private house expenses: 'points' system

Practice proportion of private house expenses

House expenses	£
Rent	–
Council tax	825
Lighting and heating	892
Repairs and renewals*	598
Window cleaning	65
Insurance	150
Domestic assistance (£10 per week)	520
Garden expenses (1/4 of £1000 – subject to negotiation)	250
	3300
Claim: one-seventh	471

*includes: £200 interior decorating; £150 electrical repairs;
£225 part (half) cost of replacement windows.

Figure 26.2   A house expenses claim

Study allowance

Where the house is not regularly used for consultations, but the GP spends time working at home, it is much less contentious to claim a 'study allowance', based on a lump-sum estimate of the additional cost to the GP of using the house for that purpose. A typical annual claim might be £1.50 per hour for 10 hours per week over 46 weeks a year, i.e. £690. Alternatively, a round sum per week could be claimed.

Capital gains tax

One factor that frequently deters GPs from making a claim for house expenses is that they have been advised that, in the event of the house being sold at a profit at some time in the future, they will be liable for CGT on a proportion of the gain realised.

This is *not* the case; in such circumstances, CGT will not be charged unless part of the house was used exclusively for practice purposes. Even if this were the case, if the doctor acquired a replacement house also used in his practice, it is likely that 'roll-over' relief could be claimed.

It is highly unlikely that a GP selling a house which has been partially used in his practice will give rise to an actual charge on which CGT is payable.

The subject of CGT on GPs' houses is extremely complex, and specialist professional advice should always be sought. No GP should be dissuaded from making a legitimate claim for house expenses merely by the prospect of having to pay CGT at some time in the future.

Other practice expenses

Apart from private use of houses, other main items included in the claim are discussed in other chapters: motor expenses in Chapter 27 and spouses' salaries in Chapter 28. However, there are many other expenses that can and should be claimed by GPs where justified.

There is some evidence of substantial underclaiming by GPs for other expenses. It is important that they are claimed fully, not only for the purpose of reducing the GP's tax liability, but also to ensure that a full record of expenses is available in practice accounts submitted to the Inland Revenue and which may be included in the sampling process from which the GP's pay award is calculated.

Other such claims may include the following.

• *Medical subscriptions.* All GPs pay their registration fee to the GMC and will subscribe also to one of the medical defence organisations. They may also be members of the BMA, RCGP and several other societies of a more specific nature within the profession. Care should be taken to see that all these subscriptions and levies are properly recorded and claimed.

- *Charitable and other donations.* Some GPs make donations of a medico-charitable nature and, provided these are of a reasonable amount, the local Inspector of Taxes will allow them against profits. Again these should be properly recorded.
- *Medical books and journals.* Although GPs receive much literature free of charge, some subscribe regularly to medical journals, as well as purchasing books for reference purposes. All payments of this nature should be properly recorded and claimed.
- *Locum fees, etc.* Many GPs make payments to locums for temporarily looking after their practice, as well as payments for deputising and relief services. In many cases, depending largely on clauses in the partnership deed, these may be made personally by the partners rather than out of partnership funds.
- *Security expenses.* As many GPs keep dangerous drugs and equipment in their houses, the necessity for expenditure on some form of security is obvious. A proportion of the cost of installing burglar alarms, their annual maintenance and the provision of security locks should be claimed for tax purposes.
- *Bank charges.* GPs often use their private bank account to some degree for practice purposes, for example by paying part of their house costs, motor expenses and other sundry items from their private account. If a charge is made by the bank for use of this account, a proportion of the charges (but not interest) can be included in the claim.
- *Cleaning and laundry.* Most of this expense is likely to be paid from the partnership, but if privately paid, the laundry of overalls, protective clothing and the like should be claimed. Claims for the cleaning of normal wear, such as suits and dresses, is unlikely to be accepted unless a particularly good case can be made. Claims for the actual purchase of such ordinary items of clothing will not be allowed under any circumstances.
- *Medical instruments.* The upkeep of medical equipment is a proper claim and all amounts, e.g. for cleaning or replacements, should be carefully listed and included under this heading.
- *Waiting room papers and flowers.* This is often included in overall house expenses and reduced accordingly. It is preferable to claim this as a separate entity if justified.
- *Accountancy fees.* Most of the practice accountancy bills will be paid from partnership funds but, if any charges are made to individual GPs for personal expenses claims, etc., these should be claimed. No claim can be made, however the bill is paid, for dealing with a GP's personal income tax return.
- *Insurance premiums.* The insurance on the house will normally be included in a house expenses claim. Motor insurance should be included in

the claim for car expenses. However, a few premiums can be included under general practice expenses; namely public liability insurance and insurance of medical and surgical equipment.

Life assurance payments do not qualify for relief, nor do payments of sickness and permanent health insurance premiums. The cost of insuring for locum cover during a period of sickness is allowable, but receipts from such policies fall into charge for tax purposes.

- *Courses and conferences.* In many cases, costs of attending courses are refunded from NHS sources and, where no net cost is met by the GP, obviously no claim can be made.

 However, other conferences attended at the GP's own expense can be claimed for, although difficulty may be experienced in having claims for major overseas conferences accepted. If the GP is accompanied by a spouse, the Inspector of Taxes is likely to insist that his or her share of the costs is excluded from the claim.

- *Private telephone bills.* In some partnerships, it is the policy of the practice that all private telephone accounts are paid from partnership funds. However, in other cases, these will be met personally and an agreed proportion of the cost of the calls should be included in the claim. This will be a matter of record and negotiation.

- *Photographic expenses.* Many GPs use cameras for medical reasons, often in connection with training purposes. This is a reasonable claim to make, although some element of private use may have to be taken into account.

- *Maintenance of approach.* The cost of maintaining the garden and surroundings of a house used for practice purposes can be claimed in several ways. Part of the cost of the upkeep of the approach to the house, to the extent that it is likely to be used by patients, is a proper claim, either by inclusion in an overall claim for house expenses, or separately.

- *Computers and technical equipment.* The use by GPs of personally owned computers, video equipment, etc., is increasing. Where such equipment is bought and retained in the GP's private house, some difficulty may be experienced in having the claim agreed, as they are likely to be used to a large degree for private and recreational purposes. If, however, such equipment were to be bought by the practice and included as a partnership asset retained in the surgery, little difficulty is likely to be encountered.

Summary

It is assumed that GPs will spend on average £24 700 on their practice expenses in the year ending 31 March 2000. This figure, which is worked out annually by the Doctors' and Dentists' Review Body, is based on GP accounts and claims submitted to the Inland Revenue, and may undervalue the total amount spent.

If a GP spends less than this, both through his partnership and by way of personal expenses claims, he may not be claiming all that he should.

27 Cars and motoring
Michael Gilbert

Virtually all GPs use their car to a greater or lesser degree for practice purposes. There is little difficulty, in principle, in obtaining tax relief on part of the expenses thus incurred. However, the proportion to be claimed is dependent on the personal circumstance of each individual GP.

Type of car

There is no restriction on the type of vehicle on which allowances can be claimed. Claims can be allowed on cars, motor cycles and even bicycles. In theory, it is not of undue concern whether the doctor runs a Rolls Royce or a Mini (but beware of the expensive cars rule); the expenses will be allowed and calculated on the same basis.

What expenses can be claimed?

The claim should include all amounts spent during the year of account in running, maintaining and servicing the car. Estimates should be avoided. Such expenses are likely to cover:

- road fund licence
- motor insurance premiums
- MOT tests
- petrol and oil
- repairs and servicing
- interest on loan finance (which may be restricted)
- hire purchase interest
- car parking
- car washing charges
- AA/RAC subscriptions
- other emergency services.

It is essential that all receipts are retained for inspection if required.

Other travelling expenses

Other forms of travel can be claimed where relevant, usually without any restriction for private use, where amounts have been specifically spent on business use. These may include such items as taxi, train and bus fares.

Calculating the 'private use' element

The most contentious part of preparing and agreeing claims of this nature is determining the element of private use which has to be taken into account before the Inland Revenue will accept the claim as allowable for income tax purposes.

Rarely are GPs' cars genuinely used 100% for practice purposes. For the most part, the car which is the subject of a claim will be used both for practice and private purposes. The Inland Revenue rule is that travel between home and surgery is considered as private use; the car that the GP uses for his rounds will almost certainly travel from home to the surgery and back at least once a day and this cannot be treated as practice use.

The Inland Revenue will dispute claims that are not prepared logically, i.e. by assuming a claim of 95% without any evidence to support this. Claims formulated in this way may be the subject of enquiries by the Inland Revenue under random audit and can result in claims for arrears of tax, interest and penalties.

To establish business mileage, it is necessary to keep detailed records of mileage for a specimen period of not less than two months, allocated between practice and private use. This can be summarised and the two factors added together to produce an agreed proportion. A typical example of the calculation of a mileage log kept for a period of two months is set out in Figure 27.1.

More than one car

GPs frequently ask whether they will be able to claim tax relief on more than one car. There is no reason why not, as long as reasonable claims are submitted, which can be substantiated in the normal manner. Major claims should be made for the principal practice car and minor claims for the second car, and an example could be:

First car	80%
Second car	30%

Dr John Wilson and his wife Mary each run a car, both of which are used to some degree in his medical practice. John has been advised by his accountants to keep a detailed mileage log for each car for a specimen period of two months in order that his proportion of private use can be accurately calculated. Both John and Mary produce weekly mileage figures which, when collated, show the following results.

Mileage logs: June/July 1999

	John [Rover] Miles			Mary [Mini] Miles		
	Total	Practice	Private	Total	Practice	Private
Week ended:						
June 7	475	420	55	63	20	43
14	125	50	75	385	195	190
21	578	300	278	75	15	60
28	487	400	87	88	8	80
July 5	569	525	44	56	16	40
12	87	20	67	468	170	298
19	625	557	68	42	24	18
26	480	404	76	50	38	12
Aug 2	360	350	10	68	34	34
Total (2 months)	3786	3026	760	1295	520	775
Percentages		79.9	20.1		40.2	59.8

From this log it would seem that John could justify a practice claim for 80% of the Rover (20% restriction) and for 40% of the Mini (60% restriction).

Figure 27.1 Mileage log for a GP's cars

If claiming for two cars, it is desirable to again maintain a regular mileage log (*see* Figure 27.1).

It is not sufficient merely to have a second car available for use as required or in emergencies; a claim can only be entirely valid if the GP can demonstrate at least some regular element of practice use.

Expensive cars

The Inland Revenue define an expensive car as one costing over £12 000.

If a car is bought for an amount in excess of this figure, the capital allowances (*see* below) are calculated as if the car had cost £12 000.

This restriction also applies to claims for interest relief on the cost of financing the purchase. This will normally be scaled down proportionately. If a GP leases a car, any tax relief he might claim for leasing charges will be similarly reduced.

Tax allowances for depreciation

GPs will be granted an annual capital allowance ('writing-down allowance') on the cost or written-down value of the car, amounting to 25% per annum.

If a car is sold, a GP will receive a balancing allowance if the sale price is less than the written-down value, or be subject to a balancing charge if it is greater.

Examples of two separate car purchases, one of these an expensive car costing over £12 000, are shown in Figure 27.2. At the end of the lives of the cars they are sold by the GP, one of them giving rise to a balancing allowance and one to a balancing charge. In the case of the expensive car, the annual writing-down allowance is limited to what it would have been had the original cost of the car been £12 000.

All claims, including the annual allowance, balancing allowance and balancing charge, will in practice be reduced by the amount of the agreed element of private use. Thus, if in our example Dr Leech has agreed he will claim 80% expenses on his 'Super Road-Hog', the allowance for the 1996/97 year of £3000 would be reduced to £2400.

The granting of capital allowances on these cars works the same way as expenses are claimed and profits assessed for tax purposes, i.e. on an accounts basis. Therefore, from the illustration, Dr Leech makes up his

	Dr John Leech	
	Bloggs Banger D436TGM	Super Road-Hog J639ABC
Accounting year-end: 30 June		
Banger, bought April 1995	7000	
Road-Hog, bought June 1995		15 500
Writing-down allowance, 1995/96 (25%)	1750	3000*
	5250	12 500
Writing-down allowance, 1996/97 (25%)	1312	3000*
	3938	9500
Writing-down allowance, 1997/98 (25%)	984	2375
	2954	7125
Banger sold: December 1997	2750	
Road-Hog sold: March 1998		8250
Balancing allowance: 1998/99	204	
Balancing charge: 1998/99		(1125)

*Restricted allowance
In practice, all claims will be reduced by agreed proportion of private use.

Figure 27.2 Capital allowances on cars

accounts to 30 June 1995 so that these would first be allowed for tax purposes in the 1995/96 tax year.

Timing of purchase

Many GPs ask what is the best time for them to change their car for tax reasons. However, there are many reasons for changing cars, not all of them financial. A car may be several years old and expensive in terms of repairs and parts; in these circumstances, it may be sensible to dispose of the car for whatever it will fetch, regardless of timing.

In general, though, a GP would be well advised to change a car immediately before his financial year-end. Again, taking the illustration, if Dr Leech wishes to change his car he should do so in June rather than July each year. This will mean that he will receive the first annual allowance for that car a year earlier. Thus, if he bought the car in June 1995 as he did, he would get the allowance in the 1995/96 tax year. Had he delayed the purchase for a few weeks and bought it in early July, he would not have received the first tax allowance until the 1996/97 year.

Financing the purchase

Few GPs can afford to buy their cars without recourse to some means of finance. There is a clear scale of preferred means of acquiring a car, the order of which is shown below.

1 Outright purchase without recourse to borrowing.
2 Free (or low) loan from motor dealer or agent.
3 Bank loan.
4 Hire purchase.
5 Leasing.

The first institution approached by a GP wishing to borrow money to finance a new car should be his bank. Hopefully, he will be regarded as a good credit risk and the bank should be able to offer a fixed interest loan, probably a business development loan, on which the interest will remain constant for the two- or three-year period. Loans of this nature should not extend to a date later than the anticipated life of the car.

Buying or leasing

There has been much comment in recent years about GPs leasing cars for use in their practice and obtaining tax relief on the premiums. Experience shows that the overall cost of leasing is likely to be greater than the monthly cost of buying a car under a bank loan or hire purchase.

It is difficult to generalise because there are numerous types of leasing contracts, many of which involve variations in payments for repairs and running costs and, above all, the conditions on which the car might be transferred to the lessee after the contract period. Each scheme must therefore be evaluated separately and considered on its merits.

GPs, by virtue of their exempt status for VAT (*see* Chapter 30), are unable to recover the VAT charged by the leasing company on the monthly charges. This greatly increases the cost to the GP and, for that reason, the leasing of cars by GPs is not generally considered to be financially viable. Some practices may, however, be able to register for VAT.

Tax saving on cars

There is likely to be a private use restriction on any tax relief claimed on cars, according to the circumstances of the GP concerned. However, provided the normal rules are adhered to, the treatment of GPs' cars for tax purposes is not ungenerous. It is worth emphasising that necessary and normal expenditure on cars can be an excellent and useful method of tax saving, as long as all expenditure is recorded, all bills are retained and a full and accurate claim is prepared. A methodical system of recording such expenditure is vital.

Finally, it is *not* financially efficient to buy and sell cars purely for the tax relief. The cost of buying a new car is far more than a GP would receive in tax relief, which should be regarded as an incidental benefit.

28 Spouses and families
Michael Gilbert

This chapter considers the financial aspects of the part which the GP's spouse and family play in his practice.

A spouse's salary

The facility for GPs to pay a salary to their spouses is an excellent if limited means of tax saving. In effect, a salary can be paid up to a prescribed level to the spouse for certain qualifying duties. This salary will qualify as a tax-allowable expense by its inclusion in the GP's own claim for personal practice expenses and, provided she has no other income, the salary will be free of tax in the hands of the recipient.

It is standard practice to maintain this salary at a level below the threshold at which Class 1 NIC (*see* Chapter 29) come into force, to avoid the payment of these contributions both by the spouse, as the employee, and the GP as the employer. The payment of such contributions would diminish any tax relief available to the GP.

For the 1999/2000 tax year the threshold at which Class 1 National Insurance comes into force is £66 weekly, which works out at £3432 per annum or £286 per calendar month. It is therefore suggested that the level of the spouse's salary be kept at a level no higher than £280 monthly.

Qualifying duties

To ensure that the payment of the spouse's salary will not be challenged by the Inland Revenue, they should be performing duties commensurate with the payment made. Those duties typically include:

- telephone answering
- secretarial and reception duties
- chauffeuring
- book-keeping, including signature of cheques
- chaperoning.

In some cases, it may be possible for other duties to be performed, depending on the spouse's professional qualifications.

Should a payment be made?

To ensure that the salary is acceptable to the Inland Revenue, a payment should be made by the physical transfer of funds, ideally as a monthly cheque drawn on the GP's bank account in favour of the spouse. Some couples, however, have joint bank accounts and in these cases it may be preferable for either a cash cheque in favour of the spouse to be drawn or for a separate account to be opened in the spouse's name and the salary paid into that account. However the salary is paid, there *must* be evidence of a physical transfer of funds.

Payment by partnerships

Partnerships frequently seek to pay out salaries of this nature to the spouses of GPs from partnership funds. This is not recommended, because it is rare for a partnership to be made up of married GPs only. Other GPs in the practice may be single. It could therefore be unfair if these salaries are paid from partnership funds and taken into account before the partnership profits are allocated. In addition, some of the partners may have chosen to pension their spouses (*see* below); it is unlikely that they will all be of the same age and attract identical pension contributions. Again, unfairness can result if pensions are paid from partnership funds.

For these reasons, it is suggested that spouses' salaries should be paid by the GP for whom they will largely be working, except in the case of spouses who work in the surgery on a regular basis.

A spouse who has outside employment

Frequently, spouses of younger GPs tend to have outside employment, and it is often assumed that in these cases a spouse's salary should not be paid. This is not the case. If a spouse earns sufficient income from their outside job to cover their personal allowance, there may be no tax benefit to the family unit concerned. This would be the case if their highest rate of income tax was equal to that of the GP. There could actually be a loss if the spouse is paying a higher rate of tax than the GP. In such a case, a salary cannot be beneficial and should not be paid. In most cases, however, a salary can be paid, if only to maintain a precedent. A spouse may choose to leave their outside employment and the salary would then become of great benefit.

Spouses' pension plans

A further means of tax saving is to take out a pension scheme for a spouse employed in the GP's practice. The premiums paid under such a policy are allowable deductions for income tax purposes and the GP will receive tax relief for them. On retirement, the pension arising from such a policy will be treated as earned income for the spouse.

The Inland Revenue has in a few cases judged the level of salary paid to the spouse on the basis of the total payment, that is to say the salary and pension premiums combined. It is therefore even more important to ensure that the salary on which the pension is based is paid for service provided at a realistic rate of remuneration paid on a regular basis.

Payments to children

A GP's family unit may include responsible teenagers who can do some of the work which the spouse of a married GP often performs, such as reception/telephone answering duties. If this is the case, a realistic salary can be paid to the children concerned.

29 National Insurance contributions
Michael Gilbert

National Insurance is sometimes called 'the hidden income tax' because it receives relatively little publicity and changes made are not normally announced in each year's Budget.

National Insurance contributions (NIC) can account for a surprisingly large slice of a GP's income. There are four main classes of insurance which may apply to a greater or lesser degree to most GPs.

Class 1 contributions

Class 1 NIC are paid by deduction from an employee's wage or salary. The rates are calculated by means of contribution tables and paid over to the Inland Revenue by the employer each month, together with the staff PAYE deductions.

Some employees may have elected to join the NHS superannuation scheme, which means that they are part of an employers' scheme and consequently pay lower contributions.

GPs, as employers, are in many cases able to recover 100% of their share of NICs for practice staff from the HA.

Class 2 contributions

Class 2 contributions are paid by self-employed people, including GPs. They can be paid by a system of quarterly billings by the National Insurance Contributions Office of the Inland Revenue who are responsible for the collection of NIC. There is also a facility for payment by direct debit, either from the personal account of the doctor concerned or from a partnership account. Such contributions are the personal liability of the doctor concerned and are not an item of partnership expenses; they should be charged to his current account.

GPs who pay Class 2 NIC by either of the above methods should ensure that they obtain credit for weeks when contributions are not payable, either through sickness or a period of unemployment.

Class 3 contributions

Class 3 contributions are paid by non-employed people, usually to protect their rights to a state retirement pension. These are frequently paid by men who retire before the age of 65 years and who have not made a sufficient contribution during their working lives to qualify for a full pension. Payment is on the same basis as for Class 2.

Class 4 contributions

Class 4 contributions are paid on a band of income which changes from year to year. In the 1999/2000 year, earnings falling within this band of income were assessed at 6% and the maximum amount which could be paid by any contributor was £1108.20.

Registration

The practice manager is strongly advised to ensure that all GPs in the practice have a National Insurance record. New partners should approach the Contributions Agency to register for this purpose, by writing to:

National Insurance Contributions Office
Class 2 Group
Longbenton
Newcastle-upon-Tyne
NE98 1YX

Deferment

Some GPs will be required to contribute to three separate classes of National Insurance: 1, 2 and 4. Classes 2 and 4 are required because they are self-employed taxpayers and Class 1 will be paid by GPs who take appointments at local hospitals. In these cases, it is possible to obtain a deferment of Class 4 and in some cases Class 2 contributions where it is evident that the GP will pay in excess of the annual maximum.

Deferment is applied for by submission of form RD1301 to the National Insurance office by 5 April in each tax year. Where deferment is obtained, but the eventual contributions under Classes 1, 2 and 4 are insufficient to meet an annual maximum figure, a demand for unpaid contributions will be issued, probably for several years in arrears.

Repayment

Where, on the other hand, contributions for a single year are overpaid, a repayment will be sent to the contributor. In the case of a partnership, it is important, to ensure fairness, that the payment is credited to the partner who paid the original contribution.

30 VAT and the GP
Ray Stanbridge

Background

Value Added Tax (VAT) was introduced in 1973 as part of the Treaty of Rome, through which the United Kingdom became a member of the Economic Community. The legislation was substantially updated in 1994 through the provisions of the Value Added Tax Act. This act, together with subsequent amendments to Finance Acts, is the basis of the current situation. The current standard rate of VAT is 17.5%.

The basic rule: medical services provided by a GP are exempt from VAT

From the outset, the supply of services by a registered medical practitioner (which for the purposes of the legislation includes dentists and allied services) is exempt from VAT as one of the several exceptions covering health and welfare services in general.

In practice, this means that a GP, regardless of his level of earnings, is not required to register or account for VAT. Under exemption provisions, a GP is not required to add VAT to fees to patients. However, he cannot recover the input tax on items upon which VAT is normally chargeable. These include:

- professional fees
- telephone charges
- petrol and car servicing costs
- supply of certain medical equipment
- equipment leasing charges
- fees for training, courses and conferences
- stationery bills
- gas and electricity bills.

For the majority of expenses in a typical GP's set of accounts, no VAT is chargeable in any event. Such expenses include staff salaries and wages, rent and rates, loan interest and charges, insurance premiums, life assurance and pension contributions.

By virtue of his tax status as an 'exempt supplier', a GP will therefore incur an extra 17.5% on the cost of a proportion of his practice expenses that cannot be recovered from any source. However, he will include the *total* cost of such expenses in his practice accounts (including tax) as items of expenditure upon which the Annual Review Body award is based. The expenditure is therefore, albeit in an indirect manner, refunded to him.

Changes in VAT rules that do affect GPs

If GPs run other businesses which do involve VAT chargeable supplies, the basic exemption rule described above does not apply.

There are a number of other changes in the legislation over the past 25 years that have affected GPs (Box 30.1). The impact of these changes is discussed below.

Box 30.1: VAT and the GP – changes in legislation

1973   VAT introduced in the UK. Supply of health and welfare services exempt.

1984   VAT extended to cover building alterations and extensions. No changes in cost-rent limits.

1998   Following a decision in the European courts, the scope of VAT extended to cover new building construction.

April
1989   VAT levied on contractors bills for new development. Separate cost-rent limits introduced.

August
1989   Self-supply rules introduced. GPs required to register for VAT in certain cases.

January
1992   Self-supply principle extended to surgery extensions.

January
1993   VAT added by FHSAs to determine cost-rent reimbursement.

March
1995   Changes in the self-supply rules.

March
1997   Self-supply changes discontinued.

Surgery development and the 'self-supply' rulings on construction prior to 1 March 1995

When VAT was introduced in 1973, no VAT charges were levied on any building work usually undertaken by GPs. In 1984, the extension in the coverage of VAT to include alterations and extensions to existing buildings did affect those GPs who were embarking on an enlargement of their surgery premises, or who were seeking to buy a property for redevelopment into a new surgery. As cost-rent limits were not extended to include the new VAT charges, GPs who did develop and renovate existing buildings were unable to claim a cost-rent limit which reflected the true amount paid.

The further extension of VAT in 1988 to cover all *new* building construction work caused further problems for GPs wishing to build new premises, since they were unable to register for VAT. However, from the date of the new ruling (1 April 1989) cost-rent limits were increased to reflect the higher costs, through application of VAT, of a new construction. No charges were, however, made to cost-rent limits in respect of building alteration work.

With effect from 1 August 1989, doctors were brought into the new self-supply charge rules. A 'self-supply' situation occurs when a person makes a supply to himself or herself. Under such a situation, for VAT purposes self-supplied goods are regarded as:

- a taxable supply made *by* the business
- a taxable supply made *to* the business.

They were treated as 'developers' for VAT purposes if they:

- constructed a building
- ordered a building to be constructed
- financed the construction of a building with a view to selling, leasing, occupying and using all or part of it.

Under the self-supply rules, developer doctors became liable to a self-supply charge if they:

- leased out any part of the building *or*
- used it in connection with an exempt business activity, including medical practice, within 10 years of completion.

There was an exemption where building costs, including professional fees and fittings but excluding bridging interest, was less than £100 000.

However, under the rules a GP normally had to register for VAT using Form VAT 1 which was available from local VAT offices. As a result, they were able to reclaim VAT on costs of development and new constructions, including professional and other fees. However, there was a self-supply charge on completion of the construction, at the rate of 17.5% total cost of construction. This included, where appropriate, costs of land purchase, together with professional fees. To a typical GP, there was a very real cost in developing new premises. Under the self-supply rules, VAT was charged on the cost of the land purchase. This was not generally recoverable by virtue of the exempt status of the GP's normal business.

Changes were introduced on 1 March 1995. A GP as a 'developer' could choose to take himself out of the self-supply provisions, provided that he repaid any input tax already reclaimed, or potentially reclaimable. In relation to other developments subject to this charge, a final charge arose on 1 March 1997, following which the self-supply charge was discontinued.

The self-supply provisions are extremely complex. Specialist VAT advice is essential for all doctors who have constructed new surgery buildings after 1 August 1989 and who are not sure of their status or potential liability.

Surgery extensions and reconstruction

The VAT self-supply rule was extended from 1 January 1992 to include some extensions of existing surgeries if the extended building were to use land outside the bounds of the previous building. If a GP (or partnership) owned at least 75% of all the land, both new and existing, for 10 years *prior* to the extension being completed, the self-supply charge rules would not apply. From January 1992, in cases where the extension or enlargement increased the surgery floor area by more than 20%, the self-supply charge was based on the cost of the works and land proportionate to the increase in floor area.

The rules from January 1992 also stated that the self-supply charge was only relevant to surgery reconstruction where the total cost exceeded £100 000, and which involved the removal or charge to 80% or more of the floor structure.

VAT and cost-rent reimbursement

There were many problems in interpretation of the impact of the new self-supply rules between 1989 and 1993 on cost-rent reimbursement. These were clarified from June 1993 where FHSAs would add VAT, as incurred, to total cost. The current situation is that:

- GPs developing *new* surgeries should add VAT to their total cost and this will then be included in their cost-rent reimbursement
- the lower rate B will continue to apply where GPs have extended or altered their surgeries.

The effect of VAT partial exemption provisions on GPs

New rules were introduced from April 1992 that allow for GP practices to be registered as 'partially exempt'. By doing this, they are able to recover an element of VAT on inputs in respect of services which they undertake outside their normal medical activities, and which are liable to standard rating.

Typical examples of income that may accrue to general practices and which could carry VAT include:

- royalties
- lecturing fees
- articles for publication
- non-medical retainer fees
- passport authentication fees
- private prescriptions
- proceeds from pay phones, coffee machines, etc.
- fees for travel packs, condoms, etc.
- advertising fees, derived, for example, from advertisements or posters in the waiting room and in practice leaflets
- PGEA meeting charges.

The rules for claims under a 'partially exempt' status were clearly defined in April 1992:

- firstly, input tax directly attributable to non-medical supplies (such as the above) is fully recoverable
- secondly, input tax directly attributable to exempt medical supplies is irrecoverable
- thirdly, the residual input tax relating to both taxable and exempt activities is partially recoverable. This must be in accordance with standard methods, or as agreed between the GP and the local VAT office.

There is, of course, a complication, through the application of the 'de minimis' rule. This provides that when the exempt input tax of a doctor is not more than £625 per month on average or £7500 per annum *and* where this input tax is no more than 50% of all input tax, all input tax shall be treated as attributable to taxable supplies, so that the doctor is fully taxable and able to recover all input tax. Output tax would, in theory, be applied, and this is contrary to the exempt status of medical work.

This 'de minimis' test must be applied for each VAT return and again at the end of each year. In practice, however, it means that consideration of exemption is only practical (and probably beneficial) to medium-sized practices, with exempt input tax of less than £625 per month. Even so, the cost of book-keeping and compliance with VAT regulations often exceeds the practical benefits.

VAT on drugs

GPs who dispense drugs from full dispensing practices or through supply of occasional items such as influenza vaccines, pay VAT to the drug supplier. Such practices are not required to register for VAT, the cost of which is effectively recovered through the standard drugs tariff.

Where a practice employs a registered pharmacist, the dispensing of drugs is subject to VAT at a zero rate. The practice can therefore register and re-claim VAT on the purchase of these drugs. Reimbursement for the cost of the drugs will, as a result, be exclusive of VAT (but *see* below).

Where a non-dispensing practice registers for VAT under these rules, the drugs administered by a GP will be part of his exempt services.

A GP can reclaim the VAT on the drugs, together with an element of VAT on costs and overheads. By undertaking this step, however, there is a danger that the 'de minimis' limit is exceeded.

General

VAT is a complex tax. As a general rule, GPs should normally be content with their exempt status. Partial exemption can, in certain individual cases, lead to some recovery of tax, but the book-keeping and compliance require-ments are generally very heavy and costly. Any recovery benefit may be off-set. The VAT treatment of buildings and building alterations is particularly difficult. It is, in practice, impossible to give anything but the most general of guidelines. Individual advice on a particular situation in this respect is essential, generally in advance of any activity taking place.

31 A look at insurance
Malcolm Dalley

One of several professional advisers the GP may consult during his working life is the insurance broker. However, many doctors do not use a single broker but buy policies on a random basis, often without any overall planning.

Constant, regular and knowledgeable insurance advice is essential for the GP, who will not only have to insure his life in the event of early death but will also find it necessary to provide cover for more mundane matters such as the house, car and surgery.

For GPs in particular, whose requirements – particularly in the form of pension provision (*see* Chapters 32 and 33) – may be very different from most other sections of the community, it is advisable, if not essential, that any insurance adviser consulted understands how GP finance works and therefore can accurately assess a GP's insurance needs.

The Financial Services Act

Introduced in 1986, the purpose of this Act is to give consumers, including investors and policy holders, a measure of legal protection that they have not previously enjoyed.

One feature of the Act is the requirement for those giving advice of a financial and investment nature to be registered under one of the regulatory bodies. Many brokers are registered with the Personal Investment Authority (PIA). Anyone seeking to take out insurance policies or deal with investment matters through such an intermediary or broker should check that the broker is a member of such a regulatory body.

A further feature of the Financial Services Act is that anyone offering such advice must do so honestly and is required, for instance, to offer a policy best equipped to meet the client's needs. For example, a client should not be advised to take out a policy merely because it pays the broker the highest commission. Indeed, the broker must, on request, disclose to a client the amount of commission he is receiving.

House insurance

A GP will need to insure his private house against such eventualities as fire, burglary and theft. Many insurance companies now offer comprehensive policies including standard cover of this nature.

Fire insurance, in particular, should be kept up to date. A GP should be aware of current property values to ensure that any award is not an underestimate in the event of a loss. The operation of the 'average' clause on insurance claims could mean that, if a householder was under-insured, the insurance company would pay out only an equivalent proportion of the claim. Many insurance companies now offer automatic adjustments to annual building costs so that the cover is maintained at the required level.

Those taking out mortgages to finance private houses will find that such insurance is normally arranged through the building society or other lender, although it is advisable to check that the premiums paid are competitive.

Surgery insurance

Every GP should ensure that full and adequate insurance of the surgery is maintained. Where a surgery is developed and a loan taken out, it is normally a condition of the mortgage that such a policy be maintained on a regular basis. In larger practices, the responsibility for dealing with surgery insurance will generally lie with the practice manager.

A GP should ensure that *all* possible losses are covered by insurance. In certain areas, this may be alleviated by efficient security procedures.

In a group practice, the cost of surgery insurance is normally treated as a partnership expense and is paid by the partners in accordance with their shares of partnership profits.

Car insurance

Virtually all GPs run motor cars and have to insure them, not only for their own protection but in accordance with the law. The insurance of motor cars on anything other than a fully comprehensive basis is not usually beneficial, except in exceptional cases or where the vehicle may not be of significant value.

Some practices are able to make savings in insurance by negotiating a 'group premium' under which all the partners' cars are insured under the same policy. There may be partnership cars used by partners or other staff which are the responsibility of the partnership, and the cost of these should fall on partnership funds.

In a partnership, it is important to establish whether the insurance premiums on the partners' own cars are to be charged against partnership profits or to be met individually by each partner. If, as is normal, the latter arrangement applies, each partner should ensure that the premium is included in his annual claim for car expenses (*see* Chapter 27).

Motor insurance is an extremely competitive market and numerous companies operate in the field. Over the years a few of them have been found to be less than professional in their dealings with policy holders and the motorist should ensure that his insurers are well-established and stable.

Members of the Automobile Association (AA) and other bodies are offered special rates, which can be highly competitive. Insuring direct through one of the Lloyds' syndicates can often provide a saving, but in any event the potential insurer is advised to obtain several quotations.

These should be judged on their merits, taking into account not merely the cover provided but the extent to which this is affected by the conditions of no claims bonuses, excess provisions, etc.

Professional insurance (defence societies)

A GP has to insure himself against claims for negligence. Indeed membership of recognised defence societies is normally included in the contracts of hospital doctors and the partnership deeds of GPs. It is also a condition of acceptance on to the list of an HA and by the local medical committee.

Reduced rates normally apply to GPs in the early stages of their careers and to some retired doctors.

Public liability policies

All practices should have, probably as part of a normal comprehensive cover, an insurance against claims by patients and others, possibly including members of staff, for injuries incurred in or around the surgery which could be held to be due to the negligence of the GP or practice. Although such a policy may form part of a larger package, a GP should ensure that cover of this type is in place.

Loss of profits insurance

Such a policy covers any loss of income that may arise from a fire or similar occurrence. Again, this is often built into a comprehensive package.

Permanent health (locum) insurance

The GP will need cover in the event of being unable to work through illness or injury. Such cover is referred to as permanent health insurance, although in the medical profession it is frequently termed 'locum insurance' because the effect of the claim on the policy will be to pay locums in the absence of the GP from normal duties.

This is a specialised market and the GP should seek advice from brokers with expertise in offering insurance advice to the medical profession.

Tax relief is now allowed in respect of premiums paid by GPs for their own locum cover, but any benefit received will be liable to tax.

Schemes set up for the benefit of practice staff are tax deductible to the partnership or employer, and will not attract extra NIC from either the employer or employee. However, if the benefit is payable to the employer, as is normally the case, it will be treated as a receipt of the business for tax purposes. This is then offset when passed on to the employee as a continuation of salary. The income benefit the employee receives will be taxed under PAYE and will be subject to normal National Insurance deductions. If the employee receives the benefit it will be taxed as a 'benefit in kind'.

Medical insurance

Some GPs may wish to insure the cost of private medical treatment should they or their families fall ill. This is frequently done through such organisations as BUPA or the Private Patients' Plan. Substantial discounts can be obtained if a group scheme is in operation.

Family income benefit

The NHS pension scheme (NHSPS) (see Chapters 32 and 33) provides relatively low benefit in the event of the death of a younger practitioner in service. A young GP is advised, therefore, to take out a policy that covers his family and will provide a continuing level of income in the event of an early death. It is sensible to provide cover, at least while any children are undergoing full-time education. It may also be advisable for a male GP to insure his wife; if she were to die and it became necessary to employ a nurse or housekeeper, the cost would be significant. Such cover is not unduly expensive and would provide the main protection against the financial effects of an unexpected bereavement.

Life insurance

It is advisable for a GP to have personal life cover in addition to that provided by the NHSPS, particularly in the early years when financial commitments to the family are at their most demanding and death benefits under the NHSPS are providing only a low level of protection.

There has been no tax relief available on new life assurance policies since 1984, except for those who are eligible to make contributions to a personal pension plan; for example, those GPs who have earnings from private consultancy work or NHS earnings in excess of their superannuable income.

Some mortgage protection policies also qualify for tax relief under personal pension plan legislation, but there are special limits and Inland Revenue restrictions on both term assurance and mortgage protection premiums. Expert advice is, therefore, essential.

Critical illness protection

Most medical and hospital personnel can now provide cover for themselves and their families against HIV infection contracted as a result of an accident during normal occupational duties, as well as a comprehensive range of other conditions, such as heart attack, cancer, paralysis and total disability. This is provided by a limited number of insurance companies only and is certainly not available on all critical illness plans.

School fees

For those families proposing to educate children privately, a popular means of financing this is through prior investment in life assurance policies specially tailored for that purpose.

However, for those who have left it too late to use a qualifying policy, which will normally have a minimum term of 10 years before maturity, other options are now available.

An innovative development by one or two banks and building societies has been the introduction of a 'draw-down' facility. This involves a remortgage to include the additional loan required to pay the total amount of school fees, together with a cheque book facility to pay the fees as and when required.

The interest payable on the total loan is at normal mortgage lending rates, and is only payable on the additional part of the loan as and when the fees are required. The loan can be repaid at the end of the mortgage term, either by the tax-free cash available under the NHSPS, with the lost pension benefit replaced by a free-standing additional voluntary contribution plan (FSAVC), or alternatively by some other savings plan.

Tax relief

Most of the premiums deriving from the types of policy set out above will be at least partially allowable for income tax purposes. It is important, however, to understand exactly how and to what extent this will be granted.

Surgery insurance

Premiums on such policies are normally included as an item of practice expense in the annual accounts and the tax relief will be granted fully as a regular item of expenditure. This will apply to fire, burglary, public liability, loss of profits and similar insurances.

Private houses

Those GPs who are able to sustain a claim for a proportion of their house expenses are normally able to include premiums on house insurance policies in such a claim and receive in effect such a proportion of the relief as has been agreed with the Inland Revenue.

Motor insurance

Similarly, all premiums on motor cars used wholly or partly for practice purposes should be included in an overall claim for car expenses (*see* Chapter 27), but will be subject to a restriction for private use agreed with the Inland Revenue.

Employers' liability insurance

All GPs employing staff should ensure they are covered for possible claims from staff members who may suffer injury or loss while at work, and may subsequently be able to show that their employer has been negligent. Such premiums are normally fully allowable for tax purposes.

32 Pensions
John Lindsay

Many GPs take an active interest in planning for retirement only in the years immediately approaching that date. This is unfortunate because the effect of any change is limited by the number of years during which benefits can accrue. A GP who plans for retirement in his early thirties is far wiser than the GP who does so in his mid-fifties. All GPs should keep their pension facilities, and the opportunity they bring, under constant review – circumstances change during a GP's working life and so needs vary; in the same way, legislation and changes in procedure determine the various arrangements available from time to time.

The NHS pension scheme

The present superannuation scheme dates back to the formation of the NHS in 1948. Fundamentally the scheme has remained unaltered, although there have been a number of radical and far-reaching amendments.

The NHSPS is divided in effect into two separate schemes. The one for general practitioners (i.e. medical, dental and ophthalmic contractors to the NHS) is based on 'dynamised' career earnings; the total earnings of the practitioner during his career are taken into account in arriving at the final pension and lump sum entitlement. The other scheme applies to officers, i.e. doctors, dentists and others employed in hospitals or other NHS services on a salaried basis. The ultimate benefits from this scheme are calculated on a 'final salary' basis and is outside the scope of this book.

It is not possible to explore all aspects of the NHSPS in a book of this size, but this chapter and the following one give an outline of the scheme, the range of benefits offered to GPs and the additional facilities available. In conclusion, further sources are specified from which the reader can obtain additional information.

Superannuable income

Superannuable income consists of all earnings of the GP as a contractor to the NHS, less an annually agreed average deduction for notional expenses. Currently, this estimated expenses element (calculated annually) is 34.5%.

There are, however, exceptions to this. While that figure is deducted from all standard items of earning, such as capitation fees, BPA, item of service fees, etc., certain other items of income, such as the seniority allowance, training grant and target payments, are fully superannuable, i.e. without making the standard deduction for expenses.

Some items are not superannuable. These include refunds, e.g. of practice staff costs and rates, and reimbursements such as the notional and cost-rent allowances. A list of fees and allowances that are wholly, partly or non-superannuable is shown in Box 32.1.

Box 32.1: Superannuable income

The NHS pension scheme GP contribution rate is 6% of superannuable income.

GP NHS income consists of three types:

Group 1 payments

Payments consisting entirely of reimbursement of expenses for super-annuation purposes:

- payments and notional reimbursements under the schemes for rent and rates, and direct payments for computing costs and practice staff
- net ingredient cost (NIC), container allowances and payments in lieu of VAT in respect of the supply of drugs and medicines
- payments under the out-of-hours development scheme (SFA 59 & 60)
- all payments, except the trainers' grant, made in respect of a GP registrar. (Payments of salary and board & lodging should be treated as the superannuable income of the GP registrar)
- payments in respect of the employment of a locum under the schemes for additional payments during sickness and confinement, for single-handed rural GPs attending training courses, and payments for prolonged study leave
- additions to BPA for the employment of an assistant, *including* the higher allowance when a principal is also receiving an addition to BPA for practice in a designated area
- associate allowance

Box 32.1: *continued*

- payments under the doctors' retainer scheme
- payments made in accordance with SFA 57: LIZ Workforce Flexibilities:
  - Type 3 IPA (SFA 57.8–57.10)
  - LIZ collaborative working allowance (SFA 57.11–57.15)
  - LIZ associate doctor payment (SFA 57.16–57.19)
  - LIZ assistants' scheme (SFA 57.20–57.22)

Group 2 payments

Payments which consist entirely of net income for superannuation purposes:

- additions to BPA for practice in a designated area
- addition to BPA for seniority
- a training grant under the trainee practitioner scheme
- inducement payments
- target payments for childhood immunisation, pre-school boosters and cervical cytology

Group 3 payments

Payments which consist partly of reimbursement of expenses and partly of net remuneration for superannuation purposes:

- dispensing fees, on-cost and oxygen therapy service rents & fees paid in respect of the supply of drugs and appliances
- BPA
- standard capitation fees
- fees for vaccination and immunisation carried out for reasons of public policy
- night consultation payments (both the annual payment and consultation fees)
- contraceptive service fees
- maternity medical service fees
- payments for treating temporary residents and for providing immediately necessary treatment

Box 32.1: *continued*

- fees for providing treatment in an emergency, for the arrest of dental haemorrhage, and where a second practitioner is required to administer an anaesthetic
- initial practice allowance types 1 & 2 only; type 3 payments to GPs in the LIZ area are non-superannuable
- rural practice payments
- PGEA
- minor surgery sessional fees
- payment for health promotion programmes and chronic disease management programmes (including payments made under transitional arrangements)
- child health surveillance fees
- deprivation fees
- registration fees
- capitation additions for out-of-hours cover (SFA 82)

The superannuable element of Group 3 income (i.e. the partly superannuable income) is reviewed annually. Currently 64.5% of this income is superannuable.

A typical calculation of annual superannuation contributions is set out in Figure 32.1, although, in practice, this is calculated quarterly throughout the year.

Method of contribution

Contributions by each GP are calculated by the HA and shown as deductions on each quarterly remittance statement. It is important, particularly in partnerships where there are differing shares, or where some partners are making additional contributions, that these deductions are reflected in drawings paid to the GPs, either monthly or quarterly.

GPs in partnership

For GPs in partnership, their contributions are usually calculated by the HA according to the profit-sharing ratios in force. It is important for

Dr A has gross income for 1998/99 from NHS fees and allowances of £45 000, with a Stage III seniority award of £5425. He is a GP trainer and receives a training grant of £5500. His superannuation contribution is calculated thus:

	£	£
Fees and allowances	45 000	
Less: Notional expenses (34.5%)	15 525	
		29 475
Seniority	5425	
Training grant	5500	10 925
		40 400
Contribution at 6%		2424

Figure 32.1   Calculation of superannuation contributions

partnerships to give their HAs full notification of each change in profit-sharing ratios at regular intervals so that these can be reflected in their superannuation deductions. Failure to do so can result in partners suffering in terms of their ultimate pension entitlement.

Contribution levels

At present, GPs who belong to the scheme contribute 6% of the NHS superannuable remuneration to the NHSPS.

In addition, the NHS makes an annual payment of 4% of superannuable remuneration for these GPs.

Contributions and tax relief

Unlike the statutory tax relief granted on contributions to the NHSPS for those in the salaried sector, that available to GPs is concessionary. It is authorised by Extra-Statutory Concession A9, and must be claimed by GPs each year, by inclusion in their self-assessment tax return.

It is important that, when the annual accounts are drawn up, the contributions are shown separately in the current accounts of each partner, rather than being shown as a deduction in calculating the partnership profits. There may be a time benefit in the tax relief being granted in this way.

Tax relief on these contributions should be claimed on the GP's personal income tax return and not by inclusion in the practice accounts or in a separate claim for personal practice expenses.

Benefits of the scheme

The benefits available to GPs who are members of the NHSPS are several and substantially more than a pension and lump sum entitlement:

- a pension which is index-linked and is calculated on 1.4% of the uprated (dynamised) career earnings of the GP concerned
- a lump sum retiring allowance, entirely free of tax, normally 4.2% of the uprated career earnings (or three times the annual pension). The lump sum will not, however, reach that figure if the GP was a married man in practice before 1972, and who has not bought the unreduced lump sum
- widow's and, in respect of service since 1988, widower's pension
- children's benefit for the GP whose career is terminated by death
- a death gratuity
- ill-health retirement benefits if a GP is obliged to cease work through illness after two or more years' service.

The NHSPS offers an attractive package for GPs, particularly for those who have younger dependants. However, these benefits can be relatively modest during the earlier years of service and the younger GP may find it prudent to take out some form of family income benefit assurance to ensure a continuing and satisfactory level of income for any surviving family.

Opting out of the scheme

Since 1988, GPs have been entitled to opt out of the NHSPS. However, it is extremely doubtful that such a course of action would be of benefit to the GP concerned. A GP contemplating this course should bear in mind the implication of relinquishing a series of valuable rights, which would be difficult and expensive to buy in the private sector, most notably the indexation of the pension, the cost of which would be enormous on the open market.

The 'dynamising' factor

The pension of a practitioner is calculated by reference to total career superannuable earnings. These will include amounts earned during the early part of a GP's career, almost certainly at much lower levels of income than those in force at the time of retirement. If no adjustment is made, a pension calculation based on these figures would produce benefits much lower than those enjoyed by an employed doctor, whose pension is based upon a 'final salary' calculation.

Table 32.1 Dynamising factors

The NHS superannuable income for each year is multiplied by the factor for that year. Each year is then added up to calculate total dynamised income.

Year ending 31 March	Uprating factor	Year ending 31 March	Uprating factor	Year ending 31 March	Uprating factor
Annual uprating factors					
1949	31.554	1967	17.616	1985	02.433
1950	31.554	1968	14.216	1986	02.266
1951	29.190	1969	13.934	1987	02.132
1952	29.190	1970	13.150	1988	01.960
1953	29.190	1971	10.958	1989	01.826
1954	29.190	1972	10.145	1990	01.691
1955	29.190	1973	09.435	1991	01.564
1956	29.190	1974	09.148	1992	01.402
1957	29.045	1975	08.368	1993	01.315
1958	29.366	1976	06.022	1994	01.295
1959	26.001	1977	05.869	1995	01.256
1960	24.858	1978	05.618	1996	01.219
1961	23.769	1979	04.331	1997	01.182
1962	23.769	1980	03.682	1998	01.143
1963	23.769	1981	03.102	1999	01.095
1964	20.848	1982	02.927	2000	01.000
1965	20.848	1983	02.770		
1966	18.955	1984	02.593		

To overcome this disadvantage, the principle of uprating or 'dynamising' was formulated, by which a factor agreed and updated each year is applied to the superannuable remuneration for each year in order to convert the amount of income in the year in which it was earned to its equivalent value at the date of retirement. Those factors currently in force are shown in Table 32.1.

GPs can get a copy of their computerised superannuable pay record from the NHS pension funds office.

It is these uprated or dynamised figures that are aggregated and upon which the calculation for final retirement benefit is based (*see* Figure 32.1).

Hospital service

Most GPs, at some time, will have worked in the hospital service – usually before embarking on general practice but also perhaps as a clinical assistant in the hospital practitioner service – or have received some form of salary from the NHS in addition to their GP income. This salary is fully superannuable; therefore GPs may accrue an additional pension based on this.

Dr X, who has practised in the NHS since 1962, retired on 30 September 1997, having purchased additional years to bring his service up to 40 years, as well as the unreduced lump sum.

His total career NHS earnings, after the operation of the dynamising factor, gives uprated career earnings of £1 700 000.

He will receive an annual pension of 1.4% of that amount, i.e. £23 800 per annum, together with a lump sum entitlement of 4.2%, or £71 400.

Figure 32.2　Calculation of final retirement benefits

To take account of this other service, depending on its length, a GP will receive either a pro rata increase of the practitioner pension or an additional officer pension in respect of hospital service. In addition, a lump sum is received which can be up to three times the annual pension.

Purchase of additional benefits

The Inland Revenue does not allow total superannuable service to exceed 45 years, of which not more than 40 may accrue before the age of 60 years.

As most practitioners qualify at or about the age of 24 years, it is not possible for more than 36 years of superannuable service to be acquired by the age of 60; in many cases, it will be less and a GP would be unable to retire on what is seen to be a full pension. For this reason, facilities have been introduced within the NHSPS for the purchase of additional service in the form of 'added years'.

The added years scheme

The present scheme for purchase of added years was introduced in the early 1980s. Its main feature is that the practitioner contracts to pay a fixed additional proportion of NHS superannuable earnings into the scheme for which extra benefits will be received, in the form of pension and lump sum on retirement.

There are two limitations.

1 Total service worked and added years purchased must not exceed 40 years at age 60.
2 The maximum total permitted contribution to the scheme is 15% of the superannuable remuneration, including the standard 6%, so that the maximum allowed payment for added years cannot exceed 9% of that remuneration.

For younger practitioners, the cost of buying their full entitlement will be considerably less than 9%, but for those of more senior years the effect of the 9% limit is likely to mean that they are unable to purchase all the added years for which they are eligible. Current calculations, in percentage terms, for purchasing these added years are shown in Table 32.2 (1).

The unreduced lump sum

Married male practitioners in the NHS before March 1972 will receive a lump sum retiring allowance for each year of service prior to that date at one-third of the rate applicable to each year subsequent to March 1972. However, a facility is available that enables such GPs to purchase the missing proportion of their lump sum. The principles and limitations of the scheme are similar to those for buying added years and the costs of this are also set out in Table 32.2 (2).

Contributions to private schemes

GPs in the NHS, both doctors and dentists, are in a unique position in that, while self-employed, they are also members of an occupational pension scheme. This unusual status provides them with opportunities not available to other self-employed people, which enable them to make private pension provision in respect of:

- non-superannuable income ('topping-up')
- superannuable earnings, if tax relief on contributions to the NHSPS is renounced
- earnings of a spouse employed by a practitioner or his practice (this is discussed more fully in Chapter 28).

'Topping-up'

A GP has the facility to pay personal pension contributions on the proportion of relevant earnings, i.e. Schedule D taxable income, derived from non-NHS sources. This process is popularly known as 'topping-up' and is calculated by multiplying the standard contribution to the NHSPS in any given year by a factor of 100/6, such product then being compared with the Schedule D income. If the Schedule D income is higher, contributions can be made to a private scheme. The method of calculation is shown in Figure 32.3.

Table 32.2　Additional NHS benefits

1 Cost of buying added years (fixed percentage to nominated birthday)

Extra % of pay required as additional contributions to buy one year of additional service – when paid from the 'Age next birthday' to the 'Chosen birthday'

Age next birthday	Chosen birthday		Age next birthday	Chosen birthday		Age next birthday	Chosen birthday	
	60	65		60	65		60	65
	%	%		%	%		%	%
20	0.50	0.36	35	0.85	0.67	50	2.25	1.38
21	0.52	0.38	36	0.89	0.69	51	2.53	1.48
22	0.54	0.40	37	0.93	0.72	52	2.86	1.60
23	0.56	0.42	38	0.98	0.74	53	3.26	1.74
24	0.58	0.44	39	1.03	0.77	54	3.80	1.90
25	0.60	0.46	40	1.09	0.80	55	4.58	2.08
26	0.62	0.48	41	1.15	0.83	56	5.77	2.30
27	0.64	0.50	42	1.22	0.87	57	7.77	2.56
28	0.66	0.52	43	1.30	0.91	58	12.06	2.92
29	0.68	0.54	44	1.39	0.95	59	–	3.40
30	0.70	0.56	45	1.48	1.00	60	–	4.10
31	0.72	0.58	46	1.58	1.06	61	–	5.20
32	0.75	0.60	47	1.70	1.13	62	–	6.97
33	0.78	0.62	48	1.85	1.21	63	–	10.42
34	0.81	0.64	49	2.03	1.29			

2 Cost of purchasing the unreduced lump sum (GPs practising before 1972 as married men)

Extra % of pay required as additional contributions to buy a bigger lump sum for one year – when paid from 'Age next birthday' to the 'Chosen birthday'

Age next birthday	Chosen birthday		Age next birthday	Chosen birthday		Age next birthday	Chosen birthday	
	60	65		60	65		60	65
	%	%		%	%		%	%
30	0.08	0.07	41	0.13	0.10	53	0.38	0.20
31	0.08	0.07	42	0.14	0.10	54	0.45	0.22
32	0.09	0.07	43	0.15	0.11	55	0.54	0.24
33	0.09	0.07	44	0.16	0.11	56	0.68	0.27
34	0.10	0.08	45	0.17	0.12	57	0.91	0.30
35	0.10	0.08	46	0.19	0.12	58	1.42	0.34
36	0.11	0.08	47	0.20	0.13	59	–	0.40
37	0.11	0.08	48	0.22	0.14	60	–	0.48
38	0.12	0.09	49	0.24	0.15	61	–	0.61
39	0.12	0.09	50	0.27	0.16	62	–	0.82
40	0.13	0.09	51	0.30	0.17	63	–	1.23
			52	0.34	0.19			

Dr A, a GP aged 47 years, who in 1998/99 had income assessable to Schedule D tax amounting to £55 000, is considering paying personal pension premiums. During the year ended 5 April 1999 he paid total superannuation contributions to the HA amounting to £3950, including added years payments of £1050.

	£
Superannuation paid: 1998/99	3950
Less: Added years and unreduced lump sum payments	1050
	2900
Grossed-up: £2900 × 100/6 =	48 333
Schedule D income	55 000
Non-superannuable income	6667
Allowable pension premiums: 17.5%	1167

Dr A therefore can pay only £1167 by way of personal pension premiums upon which he will obtain tax relief at his highest rate.

Figure 32.3 'Topping-up': calculation

In practice, most GPs with little or no income from outside the NHS are unlikely to be in a position to benefit from this.

The calculation must take into account the GP's Schedule D medical earnings from all sources, not merely those from his partnership.

Those with non-NHS earnings should make a provision for them in order to gain tax advantages and a higher total income in retirement.

Renunciation of tax relief

Relief may also be relinquished. In such circumstances, a GP may make personal pension provisions for earnings already superannuated under the NHSPS. This reduces tax relief on the payment for the personal pension by the amount of relief not claimed on contributions to the NHSPS. This is an extremely valuable option and one that should be exploited whenever possible. However, such a procedure involves any GP in a much greater outgoing from his disposable income and he must be satisfied that such expenditure will not cause undue financial difficulty. A typical calculation is shown in Figure 32.4.

A GP's decision to renounce tax relief on NHS contributions is an annual election, i.e. a GP can decide each year whether or not to pursue this course. Such an election can be made for the present year of assessment and the preceding tax year. Beyond that, retrospective renunciation is possible only for those years on which assessable income has not been finalised.

Dr B is a GP aged 58 years with NHS superannuable remuneration for 1998/99 of £50 000 and a Schedule D tax assessment of £48 000. His top rate of tax is 40%. His contribution to the NHSPS is 6% of £48 000, or £2880 per annum. If tax relief at 40% is claimed on this, his net expenditure is £1728.

Dr B decides to remain in the NHSPS but not to claim relief on his contributions and pay the maximum permitted amount to a private pension policy. His net outlay will now be:

	£
NHSPS contribution	
6% of £48 000	2880
Private premium (maximum)	
35% of £48 000	16 800
	19680
Tax relief	
40% of £16 800	6720
Total net cost	12 960

So, while the exercise results in more tax relief being available to Dr B, this is not the most significant feature. By making these arrangements, his net outlay has risen from £1728 to £12 960, by which means he has purchased additional pension benefit.

However good the potential benefits from the scheme, it is vital that the cost of their acquisition is appreciated.

Figure 32.4 Renunciation of tax relief calculation

Additional voluntary contributions (AVCs) and free-standing additional voluntary contributions (FSAVCs)

AVCs are the in-house option arranged by the NHSPS with the Equitable Life company. Low administration charges have been negotiated and no commissions are payable. FSAVCs are available through various life offices and other pension providers. AVCs/FSAVCs provide pension only without any lump sum.

At some time, a practitioner is likely to be asked to decide between buying added years, AVCs or FSAVCs, and he should be aware of the advantages and disadvantages of each, which are set out in Table 32.3. Care should be taken that any FSAVC sales person has explained the added years and in-house AVCs options. The Government Actuary has confirmed that FSAVCs are unlikely to be better value than AVCs.

The limit for contributions is the same as that for added years, i.e. a GP buying standard contributions at 6% can contribute only another 9% to the AVC/FSAVC scheme. There is a further limitation in that GPs who have already acquired – including added years purchased – entitlement to 38.1 years of pension entitlement will be unable to contribute to the AVC/FSAVC scheme.

Basic rate tax relief on FSAVCs is allowed by deduction at source. GPs who are in the higher tax bracket will obtain additional relief through their normal income tax assessments.

These, then, are the prime means by which a GP can provide for an adequate income during retirement.

Table 32.3 Added years/AVCs/FSAVCs – summary of features

Scheme feature	Added years	AVCs	FSAVCs
Contributions	Cannot vary	Variable and flexible	Variable and flexible
Benefit limits	40 years at age 60	Equivalent of 40 years at age 60 (38.1 years for GPs)	Equivalent of 40 years at age 60 (38.1 years for GPs)
GPs not claiming tax relief on NHS scheme contributions	Available	Not available	Not available
Widows'/ widowers'* and children's benefits	Available at no extra cost	Available at extra cost	Available at extra cost
Death in service/ill health benefits	Service usually enhanced	Based on size of fund	Based on size of fund
Extra lump sum	Three times extra pension	Not available	Not available
Indexing of pension	Linked to retail prices index	Available with lower pension	Possibly available with lower pension
Tax relief on contributions	Must not exceed 15% of superannuable income	Must not exceed 15% of taxable income	Must not exceed 15% of taxable income
Dependent upon investment returns	No	Yes	Yes
Dependent upon annuity rates at retirement	No	Yes	Yes
Charges and commissions	None	Low	Take care

*Widowers from 6 April 1988

33 Retirement
John Lindsay

For those approaching retirement, the prospect can be a source of considerable anxiety. Can the accustomed lifestyle of GPs be maintained on a post-retirement income? Some practitioners may be unduly pessimistic as a result of an inaccurate and/or incomplete interpretation of the inevitable financial changes that retirement produces. Unless these are identified and appreciated, a highly misleading impression of finances in retirement can result.

The three changes of greatest significance are:

- reduction in income
- increase in capital
- loss of Schedule D tax status.

Let us now look at these separately.

Reduction in income

The income reduction is often less than the GP has envisaged. This is because practitioners frequently make pointless comparisons between their NHS pension and the gross earnings it replaces. The NHS pension is taxable income and it should be related to its taxed, not gross, pre-retirement equivalent.

Another factor often ignored is the yield from investment of the NHS lump sum retirement allowance. In many instances practitioners also have some non-superannuable NHS income and earnings from private patient and/or outside sources. The latter may be from an outside appointment, insurance medicals or writing and/or tutoring. Pension provisions in respect of the taxable income from such sources is permitted and prudent GPs should make sure that appropriate pension arrangements are made for any such income. There are significant tax benefits to be gained from pensions, which can limit the reduction in income on retirement.

Increase in capital

In addition to the tax-free NHSPS lump sum and/or pension received at retirement, many GPs will have 'new' capital arising, for example from the sale of their share of practice premises, and the receipt of the proceeds from assurance policies, saving schemes and other investments tailored to terminate at retirement. If the yield from investment of these capital sums is taken into account, the earnings/pension gap can be significantly less than anticipated. It is vital that such capital is wisely invested, in order to counteract other factors, described below.

Loss of Schedule D tax status

This can have adverse implications for a retired GP. During the GP's working life, tax relief will have been obtained on certain items of annual expenditure; not all such outlay stops with retirement, but the tax saving in respect of it will cease. The extent to which this affects individual GPs varies according to their particular circumstances, but the disadvantage can be considerable.

Index-linked pensions

Working GPs have many opportunities to increase their current earnings, but once they have retired nothing can be done to alter or influence the pension payable to them.

However, index linking, offered by NHS, National Insurance and some pensions, provides extra money each year. While it does not represent a rise in real terms, index linking protects the purchasing potential of pensions. For the majority, the only real rises in retirement income will be those resulting from the adoption of a suitable investment strategy.

The lump sum

In addition to a pension, GPs receive a tax-free lump sum as part of their retirement benefit from the NHSPS. For practitioners with no NHS service before March 1972, the lump sum will be three times the initial pension. For married men with pre-March 1972 service, who have not purchased the unreduced lump sum, it will equal their pension for the years prior to March 1972 and be three times their subsequent pension. Married female practitioners, who elect to purchase a widower's pension based on their service before April 1988, will have their lump sum reduced for service during that period. However, it is possible for such a shortfall to be purchased.

It is vital for GPs to remember that their lump sum is the commuted value of part of their pension. The attraction is that, had that money been paid as a pension, it would have been taxable. The lump sum is free of tax, although the yield from its investment may or may not be taxable, depending on the sources selected. Moreover, a GP can, of course, benefit from the lump sum immediately, which may be desirable if he does not expect to live long.

Many GPs feel that their lump sum should be deposited to produce optimum instant interest or used to reduce or repay a debt. Frequently, however, neither of these courses is desirable, and it is essential that all the financial circumstances, past and future, are taken into account when the deployment of retirement capital is being contemplated.

Retirement age

GPs may only receive normal retirement benefits from the NHSPS on or after the age of 60 years, except in cases of early retirement on grounds of ill health or redundancy from a hospital post. At present, benefits can accrue up to age 70 years or until 45 years of superannuable service have elapsed.

Date of retirement

A GP should not normally retire at the end of a month as the method of calculation for retirement benefits gives a slight advantage if retirement is deferred until a few days into the following month.

Returning to work after retirement

It is possible for a GP to return to work after retirement, with the agreement of his practice partners. There needs to be a break of at least one calender month. If the GP is over age 60 there will be no abatement of pension, i.e. it is possible to retain the pension and earn income as a GP.

For those retiring before age 60 abatement applies up to that age. The pension can only be retained to the extent that pension plus NHS income do not exceed NHS income at retirement.

GPs contemplating a return to work would be wise to seek professional advice before retiring.

Post-retirement earnings

Some GPs choose to continue working after retirement, as locums, for government departments, or as medical advisers to commercial organisations. Income from these sources is taxable, and the GP is responsible for returning details of earnings to the Inland Revenue.

Provided a GP has reached the age of 65 years for men or 60 for women, he or she is not liable for any NIC arising from these earnings. However, pension contributions can be refunded on any agreed taxable profit. Such earnings, provided they are not derived from an NHS superannuable source, do not count towards the abatement of a GP's pension. However, contributions to a private pension can and should be made in respect of the taxable income from such earnings.

A retired GP is likely to require additional advice on various aspects of taxation and financial and estate planning. All these subjects can be discussed at length with a professional adviser and steps taken to obtain the maximum advantage available.

Further advice and reading

GPs who are experiencing problems in this direction or who merely require additional advice or reassurance are advised to contact John Lindsay, the head of the BMA's Superannuation Department, at BMA House, Tavistock Square, London WC1H 9JP.

BMA Services is a specialist brokerage company which provides specialist advice on the purchase of private pensions and the like. A BMA member wanting advice on these terms is advised to contact BMAS on tel: 01206 762288.

Readers wishing to obtain a fuller explanation of the subject are advised to obtain *Making Sense of Pensions and Retirement* (Radcliffe Medical Press), which considers the matter in greater depth.

34 The GP and his accountant

Although the average GP will come across many professional advisers during his working life, it will probably be the accountant who is his most regular professional adviser. A GP relies on his accountant to keep the finances of the practice and family in good order. It is a relationship that can and should be extremely rewarding on both sides, with the accountant accepted as a trusted and confidential adviser over the years, ready to offer advice at short notice. Yet the opposite is frequently the case, with the GP feeling that he is overpaying for an indifferent service. Some practices may engage four or five different firms of accountants in not many more years. Indeed, many practices may question whether they need an accountant at all.

Is an accountant necessary?

In theory, no; in practice, probably yes. A GP can negotiate taxation with the Inland Revenue and prepare his own accounts for submission and for agreement by the partners. Occasionally, single-handed practitioners may prepare their own accounts. However, in an average practice, particularly the larger partnership, the average GP has not the necessary professional skills to prepare accounts that preserve equity among the partners. Indeed, it is debatable whether any GP, after his surgical duties have been completed, would be willing and able to devote the necessary time and skill to the accounts.

Moreover, the partnership deed may contain a clause requiring the accounts to be prepared by a named qualified accountant. It is difficult to justify the removal of such a clause.

An accountant's duties

The basic duties of the accountant are to prepare the annual practice accounts and agree these with the Inland Revenue. He will also recommend payments of tax, submit computations for agreement and deal with allocations of tax payments and repayments. These are sometimes referred to as 'compliance' matters, since they largely represent legal requirements which must be complied with. In many practices, the accountant will also be called on to advise on a range of peripheral matters, such as drawings calculations, tax reserves, surgery developments, pensions and retirement, and provision of management information.

An accountant will deal with the self-assessment tax returns of both the partnership and individual partners, prepare their personal expenses claims, as well as advising on other aspects of their personal finances.

Judging an accountant's competence

Is he doing his job properly, and how can we tell if that is the case? It is notoriously difficult for one professional to judge the competence of another. However, it is possible to lay down a few general rules by which a GP can form an opinion as to whether the accountant is doing a good job.

- Are the accounts delivered within a reasonable time after each year-end? If not, it may be the result of lack of information being given to the accountant; if it can be established that the accountant is at fault, he should be made to understand that much of the value of accounts of this nature lies in their prompt production and delivery.
- Do the accounts give an idea of the manner in which income is generated and expenses paid? Do they show exactly how the profits are allocated among the partners and do they give the level of management information that will enable the practice to be run economically and efficiently? A specimen set of such accounts is shown in Chapter 10, while Chapter 12 interprets statistics which can be extracted from these.
- Is he a specialist? Does he have a copy of the Red Book available for easy reference and can he discuss with you aspects of finance exclusive to GPs, such as pensions and superannuation, cost-rent schemes, practice allowances, leave advances and item of service fees?

  It is possible for accountants to purchase the Red Book, so all accountants presuming to act for doctors should possess a copy.
- Is he efficient? Are letters answered reasonably promptly and are telephone calls returned?

The specialist accountant

Considerable benefits can be gained by a GP who engages an accountant with experience in dealing with several similar practices and who has made work for GPs his speciality. As this is crucial to the quality of service offered, any GP or practice wishing to engage an accountant should seek to confirm that a prospective accountant is a specialist. Frequently, this can be done only by personal recommendation.

For many GPs it has been easier said than done to find an accountant with the requisite level of speciality and experience which will enable him to perform the work required. Fortunately, in recent years an organisation has been set up which attempts to cater for this need.

The Association of Independent Specialist Medical Accountants (AISMA) is an association of specialist accounting firms which are accredited with work for GPs and have all satisfied the entry requirements laid down by AISMA. AISMA has produced a members' charter which is available on request and will give broad details of the level of service which will be provided by member firms. GPs wishing to make contact with an AISMA member firm should ring the Secretary (Ms Liz Densley) on 01424 730345.

Fees

The judging and evaluation of accountancy fees is probably one of the most misunderstood aspects of the accountant's function. Such fees tend to increase at a steady rate, mainly due to the competitive salaries required to be paid to staff within the accountancy profession. These increases may at times be in excess of the rate of inflation.

Most accountants charge fees by means of an hourly rate which is applied to the number of hours spent on each particular client's work, with regard to the seniority of the person involved. It is incumbent on an accountant to employ on each client's affairs the least expensive person possible without any loss of efficiency. For instance, the routine work of agreeing and balancing a petty cash book can be performed by a junior clerk.

However, the rates applied vary not only within an accountancy firm, but between different firms and in different parts of the country. In general, for instance, higher rates are applied in the South East than in the North of England or Scotland.

The vogue for judging fee levels at a fixed charge per partner for a practice should be discouraged. This is inequitable and frequently not precisely defined, in that such quotations rarely set out whether the fee includes that for the partner's personal work and for VAT. In addition, it presupposes that the cost of dealing with an eight-doctor partnership will be twice that of dealing with a four-doctor practice. This is highly unlikely; the cost may be rather higher, but certainly not double. Indeed, there is a substantial economy of scale in dealing with the larger partnerships. The cost per partner tends to reduce significantly with the number of GPs in a particular practice.

Accountancy fees vary according to numerous factors that cannot always be foreseen: the quality of records given to the accountant; the frequency of partnership changes; whether there are Inland Revenue enquiries into the practice tax affairs; the level of personal work required by individual partners; and other matters.

It is difficult to give hard and fast parameters for the level of accountancy fees which should be charged. Most quotations for accountancy fees will exclude VAT, so that an addition of 17.5% must be added to any estimate received. Thus, if a firm offers to deal with the affairs of a partnership for, say, £3000, then the actual cost of that inclusive of VAT will be £3525. As GPs are normally unable to register for VAT, this is effectively an additional cost to the practice.

In addition, regional variations come into play. Having taken all these matters into account, however, provided a practice's books are properly presented and balanced, then a charge of £1000 per partner, exclusive of VAT, would appear to be a reasonable level of fee.

A quotation of this type would normally include all the routine work of dealing with the partnership and the individual partners, but exclusive of VAT. Any additional work may have to be negotiated separately.

Personal or partnership accountant?

In partnerships, confusion often arises over whether partners should engage the same accountant who deals with practice affairs to deal with their personal finances.

If a GP has confidence in the partnership accountant, there are many advantages in using the same firm – there should be savings of costs due to minimising correspondence and telephone calls and a single accountant can obtain an overview of the practice affairs which might not otherwise be possible.

Small or large firm?

One decision the doctor will have to make on engaging an accountant is whether he wishes to use a small or large accountancy firm. There are advantages associated with both and it is important that these are appreciated.

Although the small firm may offer a less expensive and more personal service, it may not offer the level of speciality a GP requires and problems can arise when partners/principals retire or are away through periods of holiday or sickness.

A large firm will probably be able to offer a degree of speciality and the accounts will be constantly reviewed by several individuals before the work is completed. This process of review and checking so common in larger firms may increase the fees but it is in a client's interests. However, a GP may feel that in a larger firm his individual requirements are not always catered for and that a less personal service is provided.

Ultimately, it is for each GP to decide. Before making a final decision he should interview various firms. It is worth remembering that, apart from the normal professional duties, an accountant should offer peace of mind and a GP can feel secure in the knowledge that his finances are in good hands and there is no cause for worry when letters, assessment notices and the like arrive from the Inland Revenue.

35 The GP and his solicitor
Michael North

Question: 'What have you got when a lawyer is buried up to his neck in the sand?'
Answer: 'Not enough sand.'
Question: 'What is black and brown and looks good on a lawyer?'
Answer: 'A Dobermann pinscher.'
Question: 'Why do they bury lawyers 12 feet under?'
Answer: 'Because deep down they are good people.'

Lawyers do generally have a bad press and many GPs seek to arrange their affairs without recourse to specialist legal advice. In many cases, the practice accountant or banker, the HA manager or a BMA industrial relations officer will have the necessary expertise to assist the practice, but there are areas in which only expert legal advice is sufficient and it is worth investing in good advice at the outset to avoid expensive problems later.

Unlike the practice accountant, who should be involved in the day-to-day running of the practice and be consulted on the majority of financial decisions, there is no need for the practice solicitor to be so closely involved.

However, there are benefits in getting to know your solicitor and keeping him informed of major decisions so that if and when his advice is required, he is familiar with the practice and its way of working without the need for lengthy explanations. This easy relationship makes a quick consultation in advance of some actions much easier. For example, if you are considering taking disciplinary action against an employee, it is worth a telephone call to your solicitor to ensure that you deal with the matter without breaching the employment legislation or your own employment contracts. An idea of the likely consequences in terms of litigation, costs and compensation will enable you to make an appropriate and economic decision.

Solicitors should usually be involved in relation to:

- employing or dismissing staff and associated matters
- regulation of the partnership (ideally by partnership deed), including the introduction of new partners and the retirement of partners

- surgery premises
- the cost-rent scheme.

Most of these topics are dealt with in detail in other chapters of this book.

The important thing to remember is that there are many special rules which apply only to medical practitioners, and it is therefore essential that you choose a solicitor who is familiar with these rules and who has experience in advising medical practitioners. Beware, however, of allowing a specialist in one area of the law to advise you on other matters. You should find a firm that has experts in all areas of the law that you may need. If this is not possible, a firm which has most areas covered can consult other specialist firms or counsel on specific matters to ensure you receive the best advice and that the relationship between you is maintained. Switching professional advisers too frequently merely leads to time and money wasted in covering old ground again and again, but bad advice is sometimes worse than no advice at all!

Fees are often a vexed question and solicitors do tend to be viewed as expensive luxuries. However, all solicitors are required to give advance indication of how their fees will be calculated and an idea of the likely total. Many solicitors still calculate fees on an hourly rate, but fixed fees for a task are becoming more common. Remember that a specialist solicitor may appear more expensive on hourly rates, but should take less time in researching the specialist rules for medical practitioners and is therefore a better investment. If you build a good relationship with your practice solicitor and involve him in the decision-making process, you may be able to negotiate an annual retainer to cover the majority of the advice given which assists you in your financial planning.

The crucial thing in all dealings with the law is to take professional advice early enough. However much you may wish to save money on fees, problems do become aggravated through delay, and if matters deteriorate so far that litigation is necessary, the costs could rise in leaps and bounds. The earlier a problem is looked at, the easier it can be to resolve for a lawyer who knows what he is doing; so it is sensible to appoint a practice solicitor and involve him from day one.

Appendix A:
Fees and allowances for GPs, 1999/2000

		From 1 April 1999 to 31 March 2000 £
Practice allowances		
Maximum for:	BPA: full rate	8256
Designated area:	Type I	4000
	Type II	6105
Seniority:	Stage I	510
	Stage II	2700
	Stage III	5750
	Stage IV	7000
Post-graduate education allowance (full rate)		2590
Trainee supervision grant		5645
Assistant's allowance:	Ordinary	7155
	In designated area	10 015
Associate allowance* (max: 3rd year)		33 965
Leave advance (20% of BPA)		1651.20
Out-of-hours allowance		2380
Capitation fees		
Standard		
Age:	To 64	17.65
	65–74	23.25
	75 and over	45.05
Addition for out-of-hours		
Deprivation payments:	High level	11.60
(per patient)	Medium level	8.70
	Low level	6.70
New registrations		7.80
Child health surveillance		12.75
Rural practice: unit payment		0.219p

Target payments (maximum per doctor) £

Childhood immunisations:	Higher	2580
	Lower	860
Pre-school boosters:	Higher	765
	Lower	255
Cervical cytology:	Higher	2865
	Lower	955

Sessional payments

Health promotion clinics Per band (annual fee)	2480
Asthma and diabetes care (each)	435
Minor surgery (per session)	128.25

Item of service fees, etc.

Maternity fees** (obst. list: complete service)	205.00

Out-of-hours consultation   Fees per patient

Anaesthetic fee		23.80
IUCD		54.70
Contraception: annual fee		16.40
Emergency treatment and minor ops*		25.90
Temporary resident:	To 15 days	10.40
	Over 15 days	15.60
Vaccination:	Lower	6.25
	Higher	4.30
Locum allowance in sickness (weekly maximum)		491.60

*   Please refer to detailed fees as published from time to time.
** A full scale of maternity fees, depending on whether or not the doctor is on the obstetric list, is available from most medical journals.

More complete details and updated information on current rates of fees and allowances can be obtained monthly from the main medical journals: *Medeconomics*, *Financial Pulse* and *Money Pulse*.

Appendix B:
Cost-rent limits and allowances

To work out figures for potential projects, do the following calculation using the schedules below, which outline cost-rent limits for basic building and additional facilities. Multiply building cost allowance plus car park or externals allowance plus (additional facilities space approved by HA to maximum shown below multiplied by rate per m^2) by building cost location factor (contact HA) and add professional fees at rate shown. Add VAT at appropriate rate plus local authority planning permission/building regulations fees (inc. VAT) plus off-site costs, e.g. gas, electricity, water supply to site boundary (inc. VAT). Schedules apply as of 1 April 1999. GPs in the process of agreeing projects with their health authorities who have not reached tender acceptance may ask the HA to review the written offer.

Basic limits by practice size

Number of GPs	Gross internal area (m^2)	Building cost allowance ($\pounds$)	Car park ($\pounds$)	Building cost allowance for additional facilities (per m^2)	Professional fees (%)
1*	148	130 681	9027	832	12.5
2*	239	206 780	16 794	804	12.4
3*	348	287 078	23 722	753	12.3
4	476	357 929	29 705	737	12.2
5	540	399 915	34 953	726	12.1
6	600	437 702	38 837	717	12
7	654	469 191	41 986	707	11.9
8	711	501 206	44 610	698	11.8
9	771	534 270	47 234	689	11.7
10	835	568 908	49 543	682	11.6

Exceptionally, HAs may allow for extra costs for external security, e.g. shutters, glazing.
*1-, 2- and 3-GP premises are assumed to be single storey (known as type A); premises for more GPs are assumed to be two storey, with two staircases and one lift.
Exceptionally, HAs may add 35m^2 for one staircase and lift and increase cost allowance to £327 489 for 3-GP premises built on two storeys.

Limits for additional facilities

Practice manager	14 m^2 for one GP; no limit for larger premises
Part time GP	18 m^2
GP trainer: extra space	4 m^2
GP registrar	18 m^2
Dispensary	14 m^2 (1–2 GPs); 23 m^2 (3–5 GPs); additional space at HA discretion for larger premises
Services management	16 m^2 (1–2 GPs); 24 m^2 (3–4 GPs); 32 m^2 (5–6 GPs); 40 m^2 (7–8 GPs); 48 m^2 (9–10 GPs)
Services development	16 m^2 (1–2 GPs); 34 m^2 (3 GPs); 44 m^2 (4 GPs); 54 m^2 (5–7 GPs); 69 m^2 (8–10 GPs)

Appendix C:
Tax relief on pension contributions

Inland Revenue extra-statutory concession on doctors' and dentists' superannuation contributions

The following is an extract from the Regulations.

Under FA 1970, s 22 (for 1973/74 onwards; ICTA 1970, s 209 for years to 1972/73) contributions required to be made in pursuance of a public general Act of Parliament by the holder of an office or employment towards the provisions of superannuation benefits may be deducted in assessing his emoluments. These sections are in practice treated as extending to assessments under Schedule D on the profits of a medical or dental practitioner who is required to make superannuation contributions in pursuance of the National Health Service Acts. Where, however, the practitioner also pays premiums or contributions towards a retirement annuity within ICTA 1970, s 226 a restriction is imposed either on the amount of the deduction for his statutory contribution or on the amount of retirement annuity relief allowable.

For 1980/81 onwards concessionary relief is allowable on either of the following bases.

Either practitioners may have relief on the amount of their NHS contributions together with relief on the amount of any retirement annuity premium in relation to their non-NHS earnings. For this purpose:

(i)   non-NHS earnings are taken as the amount of net relevant earnings (as defined in Sec 227(5)) less the sum produced by multiplying the amount of the NHS contributions by $16\frac{1}{3}$.
(ii)   retirement annuity relief will be allowable within the normal limit of $17\frac{1}{2}\%$ (or the higher percentages for older contributors) of the non-NHS earnings plus any unused relief for earlier years. For this purpose unused relief should be calculated on the appropriate concessional basis for years in which relief has been allowed on NHS contributions.

Or, practitioners may have relief on the same basis as set out in 2 relating to the years 1972/73 to 1979/80.*

Finally, practitioners may, instead, have relief on a statutory basis. In this case, they would take retirement annuity relief, up to the limits appropriate for a particular year, on their full net relevant earnings (i.e. including NHS earnings). But in that event no concessionary relief would be available in respect of NHS contributions.

Source   IRI (1970) as amended and updated by each of the Supplements 1971 to 1975: 1977 and 1978 Supplements to IRI (1976) and amended to present wording by 1981 Supplement to IRI (1980).

Notes   In view of the number of changes that have been made to this concession
         (see sources above), careful consideration should be given to the exact
         form of the concession for earlier years.

"2   Alternatively, practitioners may have relief on the amount of their NHS con-
      tributions together with relief on any retirement annuity premiums paid up to
      the amount of the largest premium on which tax relief was allowed for any of
      the three years 1969/70 to 1971/72 – but with a restriction, if necessary, to
      keep the total relief on NHS contributions and retirement annuity premiums
      within the pre-1971/72 limits for retirement annuity relief at 10% of net
      relevant earnings of £730 – or the higher limits permitted to older people. Any
      surplus of premiums paid over the amount allowable on this basis will not be
      available for carry-forward.

         The Finance Act 1980 removed the ceilings on premiums payable and
      introduced carry-forward.

Index